T0327682

COPARTICIPANT PSYCHOANALYSIS

Toward a New Theory of Clinical Inquiry

COPARTICIPANT PSYCHOANALYSIS

*Toward a New Theory
of Clinical Inquiry*

JOHN FISCALINI

Columbia University Press   New York

Columbia University Press
Publishers Since 1893
New York   Chichester, West Sussex
Copyright © 2004 Columbia University Press

Library of Congress Cataloging-in-Publication Data

Fiscalini, John.
  Coparticipant psychoanalysis : toward a new theory of clinical inquiry /
John Fiscalini.
      p. cm.
  Includes bibliographical references and index.
  ISBN 0–231–13262–X (cloth : alk. paper)
    1. Clinical psychology. 2. Psychoanalysis. 3. Inquiry (Theory of knowledge)
    I. Title.

RC467.F54   2004
616.89'17—dc22   2004049340

∞

Columbia University Press books are printed on permanent and durable acid-free
paper.

Printed in the United States of America

c 10 9 8 7 6 5 4 3 2 1

To Barbara

Contents

Preface

Two clinical models have been dominant in psychoanalysis: first, the classical paradigm, the view of the analyst as an objective mirror. The interpersonal turn in psychoanalysis led to a second view of the analyst as an intersubjective participant-observer. Participant-observation, in its broadest sense, refers to the clinical perspectives of interpersonal psychoanalysis, self-psychology, relational analysis, intersubjectivity theory, social constructivism, and some aspects of contemporary Freudian analysis, all of which, despite their many differences, share a clinical focus on the analysis of the interpsyche (the social mind).

However, an evolutionary shift in psychoanalytic consciousness has been taking place. A newly emerging, or more accurately, reemerging third paradigm, *coparticipant inquiry*, represents a shift in analytic clinical theory. This is a major shift, with profound clinical implications (which are examined throughout the book). Coparticipant inquiry, as a unique form of clinical participation, is marked by a radical emphasis on patients' and analysts' analytic equality, emotional reciprocity, psychic symmetry, and relational mutuality. The concept of coparticipant inquiry builds upon and extends the concepts of inquiry of the two previous models of psychoanalytic praxis.

This book draws upon and is developed from arguments advanced in Fiscalini (1988, 1990, 1991, 1994a,b). Part 1, in particular (chapters 1–3), is a study and exploration of coparticipant inquiry as an evolving clinical paradigm. My aim is to delineate its salient characteristics and to articulate its radical advantages over the other models of analytic therapy. Coparticipant inquiry integrates the individualistic focus of the classical tradition and the social focus of the participant-observer viewpoint, forming, as it were, a third clinical paradigm.

Coparticipant inquiry avoids a reductionistic biological individualism (the isolated individual mind or the intrapsychic), which fails to take sufficient account of the clinical role of object relations or interpersonal relations. It also avoids the reductionistic social determinism of the participant-observer tradition in clinical work (the intersubjective mind), which has failed to take sufficient clinical account of human agency, will, and personal responsibility.

Coparticipant inquiry integrates the dialectic of human singularity and human similarity in a way that participant-observation and classical paradigms do not. Further, whereas the clinical emphases of the classical and participant-observation paradigms have been, respectively, on the impersonal and the interpersonal, coparticipant inquiry focuses on the personal.

This book traces the evolution of coparticipant practice in psychoanalysis, clarifies its singular properties, delineates its core principles, and explores its clinical implications. This necessitates a fresh look at the concept of the self. In particular, I address the clinical and theoretical implications of a dialectical relationship between various aspects of a proposed five-dimensional self. This multidimensional concept of the self is an attempt to reconcile the antinomy or paradox that mankind is simultaneously communal and individual—both embedded in a series of social fields of experience and behavior and yet also always uniquely individual. All of us are both part of others and yet also apart. Coparticipant inquiry deals with the dialectic and paradoxical nature of the self in a more comprehensive fashion than either classical theory or participant-observation. This question of the self and its clinical dialectics is examined in part 2 (chapters 4–5).

Narcissism, or the perversion of the self, is explored in part 3 (chapters 6–9). I define narcissism in the broadest sense as a complex of dynamic processes that characteristically involve or impact upon some aspect of selfhood. In my opinion, the dynamism of narcissism represents a core dimension of all psychological disorders—a kind of master neurosis—rather than a discrete diagnostic entity. As the clinical expression of self-pathology, narcissism is, in a sense, the self gone wrong. The study of narcissism thus gives us a particularly advantageous way to examine the coparticipant analysis of the self, particularly of those dimensions of the self I call the personal and interpersonal selves. The study of the clinical dialectics and coparticipant treatment of these opposed aspects of the self forms one of the central themes of the book. I see the study of narcissism, arguably today's dominant psychopathology, as integral to the central concern of the book: the study of the self and its coparticipant inquiry.

The last and largest section of the book represents some of my ideas about the nature and problems of psychoanalytic therapy. Part 4 (chapters

10–13) covers a range of clinical subjects, many of which touch upon current controversies in psychoanalytic praxis. In this part of the book, I examine the interpretation-relationship controversy as to how psychoanalysis works, and I propose that a "living through" process is essential to psychoanalytic growth. I also discuss what I call "openness to singularity," a set of attitudes and abilities that are essential in promoting analytic vitality and viability. There is also a chapter on transference analysis and one on the "analytic work space."

Various questions and controversies are visited in the chapter on transference, including questions of the nature of psychoanalytic knowledge, analytic authority, the place of authenticity in analysis, the role of unconscious communication, the question of transference as an interpersonal phenomenon, modes of listening in psychoanalysis, the question of truth, and working with human uniqueness.

The notion of an active, spontaneous coparticipant inquiry has long appealed to me. In my analytic training I found myself drawn to the freedom of interpersonal psychoanalysis rather than to the Freudian clinical model with its narrow strictures (though I was drawn to Freud's own, freer, way of working). At the same time, I was also aware of a division in interpersonal thinking between those analysts who, like Fromm, focused clinically on individual will and responsibility and defined the analytic process as a human encounter and those interpersonal analysts, who, like Sullivan, saw themselves as experts in interpersonal relations and whose clinical mandate was to carefully attend to the vicissitudes of the individual's socially determined anxiety and psychopathology. Both of these forms of participant-observation have much to recommend them. Both are in many ways compelling; yet each is seriously flawed. Fromm's approach runs the risk of becoming an authoritarian therapy that is exhortatory and blaming, that asks too much of the patient. On the other hand, Sullivan's negation of unique individuality leads to a clinical denial of the therapeutic role of personal agency, will, choice, and similar aspects of free will.

This antinomy is in some ways echoed in the debate between the followers of Kohut and those analysts who advocate a more confronting approach, as does Kernberg. These therapeutic antinomies, at the time, seemed irreconcilable, except in reductive terms. Yet I found both approaches compelling, both of them truthful and helpful. Similarly, I found obvious merit in Freud's counsel of analytic reserve, but at the same time, I was inexorably drawn to the spontaneity, aliveness, egalitarianism, and openness to self-exploration of Ferenczi's radical analytic experiments.

Coparticipant inquiry accepts this paradox and acknowledges the therapeutic potentials of both perspectives. Not unlike contemporary physicists' acceptance of the paradox of light being both wave and particle

(photon), one can, from a pragmatic perspective, enjoy the practical benefits of accepting both clinical approaches, Frommian and Sullivanian, as
offering clinical truth and benefits.

The concept of coparticipant inquiry, with its dialectical focus on both
the personally unique and the interpersonal, has affirmed and informed my
clinical experience. The principles of coparticipant analysis (outlined in
chapter 2) represent the ideals and concepts informing my own practice. I
find the following clinical emphases or features of coparticipant inquiry
particularly helpful and instructive:

1. the egalitarian emphasis on the analytic equality of patient and analyst—the nonauthoritarian acceptance of the patient as a true partner;

2. the acceptance of the patient as both a communal and a uniquely
individual being. Both the reality of personal responsibility and the need
for interpersonal responsivity are taken into clinical account. The patient
is neither seen reductively solely in terms of his or her social surround nor
studied without reference to the interpersonal context of his or her experience.

3. the bidirectionality of coparticipant inquiry, which makes possible a
freer and wider range of acceptable analytic behavior;

4. the call for greater freedom in analytic technique allows for and, in
fact, demands that as analyst I be in touch with my immediate experience;

5. the notion of the therapeutic process as a personal encounter, which
encourages greater authenticity in analytic relatedness;

6. the emphasis on there being no one "right" answer to clinical questions is a relief to us since we are so often burdened by notions of the
proper or "correct" understanding of clinical events.

These are some of the therapeutic benefits to be found in coparticipant
inquiry. This, then, takes us directly to the study of this clinical paradigm
and its evolution in psychoanalytic praxis.

Acknowledgments

This journey into the world of coparticipant inquiry was not taken alone. I would like to thank those who helped me. I would first like to thank my wife and colleague, Barbara Suter, for her love and encouragement, and her invaluable help throughout. I deeply appreciate her clinical acumen, wise counsel, and always kind critiques. For her unselfish gift of time for me to write, I am grateful beyond words. I especially want to thank her and my daughter Kate for reminding me that writing about life is not the same as living it.

I would also like to thank my friend and colleague Stanley Renshon, whose warm encouragement, thought-provoking questions, and incisive critiques of early drafts helped me to sharpen my thinking and to clarify my ideas. I also wish to thank Anthony Bass, Elizabeth Goren, and Bernadette Hogan, whose own work embodies the best of coparticipant inquiry, for their insightful commentary and critique, unstinting encouragement, and for their friendship.

I wish also to thank all those students and supervisees who have taught me at least as much as I taught them. My appreciation, too, to those who were my teachers, especially Janet Jeppson and the late Ellen Dolganos and Earl Witenberg. Special appreciation is due to my patients who have taught me much about life, and about the resilience of the human spirit.

More than anyone else, Benjamin Wolstein, now gone, helped me see the coparticipant nature of the human psyche and its psychoanalysis. His personal integrity and decency, genuine humility, creative ways of listening, and belief in the benefits of long-term psychoanalytic self-exploration continue to inform my work and to encourage my trust in my unique individuality and that of others.

At Columbia University Press, I want to thank John Michel for his graciousness, editorial expertise, and his careful shepherding of this project. I also want to thank Sabine Seiler for her keen eye and deft pen; Roy Thomas for his editorial skill and generous spirit; and Liz Cosgrove for her elegant book design.

The major task . . . will be to explore the unconscious, to investigate the subsoil of the mind.

   —Henri Bergson, *La Rêve* (1901)

There is no limitation in the here and now of the encounter between patient and analyst. When this encounter takes place, during the analytic session, when the two talk to each other, then there is nothing more important in the world.

   —Erich Fromm, *Zen Buddhism and Psychoanalysis* (1960)

It takes two people to speak the truth, one to speak, another to hear.

   —Henry David Thoreau, *A Week on the Concord and Merrimack Rivers* (1849)

COPARTICIPANT PSYCHOANALYSIS

Toward a New Theory of Clinical Inquiry

Psychoanalytic Paradigms, Clinical Controversy, and Coparticipant Inquiry

Throughout its history, psychoanalysis has been threatened by internal dissension and external rejection. In our own day, the search for psychic truth and personal wisdom in self-exploration finds a cold reception in an increasingly narcissistic, unreflective, and hurried society—impatient, addicted to magical solutions, other-directed to the extreme. Externally beset by these societal demands for an instantaneous, effortless, and painless therapy and internally split by sectarian divisiveness, psychoanalysis is now again, as in its earliest days, characterized by clinical controversy and wide differences of opinion on what constitutes the core of clinical psychoanalysis or best defines the psychoanalytic method.

Contemporary answers to many of the pressing clinical questions and theoretical issues in psychoanalysis are diverse despite recent signs of a growing rapprochement among the various psychoanalytic schools. Frequent calls for a less fractured relationship between competing psychoanalytic methodologies and metapsychologies have not yet led to greater harmony. Today, psychoanalysis, with its various subschools and clinical orientations and almost endless variety of clinical methods, goals, and practices, truly encompasses, in William James's terms, a pluralistic universe of clinical theory and method.

The psychoanalytic search for self-transformation and a healing therapy has not only resulted in a diversity of points of view; all too often it has been accompanied by political strife, rigidity of belief, and fear and contempt for innovative clinical conceptions and treatment approaches. Such narrow partisanship and diversity of therapeutic orientations is perhaps not surprising given the emotional intensity and deeply personal nature of clinical analytic work and the crucial life issues at stake for both analyst and patient. Positions taken on various clinical issues are not simply an abstract matter. They are matters of vital significance. Different conceptions of the nature of psychoanalytic data, process, method, and therapeutic action and competing metaphors of the analyst's therapeutic role—whether the analyst is seen as interpretive surgeon, objective mirror, mirroring self-object, participant observer, confronting expert, comforting supporter, participant, or coequal explorer— have very real and significant consequences for analysts and patients.

Paradoxically, despite such divisive partisanship in psychoanalysis there has been a significant cross-fertilization of ideas and practices among the different psychoanalytic schools, perhaps more so today than at any previous time in the history of psychoanalysis. Furthermore, there has been a growing heterogeneity within the various analytic schools as well as cognate developments among them. This has lead to a blurring of the boundaries between the different schools, sometimes making it difficult to know what exactly distinguishes one from another.

As our psychoanalytic universe has evolved and expanded and become ever more diverse and complex, theorists have tried to impose order on this complexity by formulating comprehensive metamodels of analytic theory and practice. Analysts from different analytic orientations have constructed meta-metapsychological schemata and meta-methodological paradigms. Thus, for example, Thompson (1950), Munroe (1955), and Hall and Lindzey (1957), writing from different psychoanalytic or psychological perspectives, advance classificatory schemas that divide psychoanalytic theory and practice into two incompatible models: the drive (libido) and the relational, cultural-interpersonal, or social-psychological (nonlibido) schools or paradigms. More recently, Greenberg and Mitchell (1983), representing a relational perspective, similarly divide psychoanalytic theory and practice into two metamodels: the relational and the drive paradigms.

Writing from a more clinical perspective, the seminal interpersonalist Wolstein (1977) states that psychoanalytic inquiry has moved from a biological (id) model to an ego-interpersonal or sociological (ego) model and that we are now moving into a third, psychological, model of psychoanalysis and to a coparticipant model of clinical inquiry. From another interpersonal point of view, Levenson (1972, 1991), employing a different clinical typology, asserts that we have moved from the machine age of Freudian analysis through the information paradigm of Sullivanian analysis into the "organismic" global time and sensibility of contemporary psychoanalytic inquiry. Similarly, Kohut (1977), writing from his unique vantage point of psychology of the self, asserts that we live in the age of tragic, rather than guilty man, and that our work is to restore developmentally arrested selves rather than to solely interpret psychic conflict. Again, there is a bifurcation of libido versus nonlibido paradigms of psychoanalytic praxis. Gedo and Goldberg (1973) call for a more complex typology or paradigmatic schema, asserting that analysts must use five different clinical models in order to understand all of their different patients.

Contemporary psychoanalysts draw primarily from three clinical models: (1) the nonparticipant mirror; (2) participant observation; and (3) coparticipant inquiry. In this book, I focus primarily on an exploration of coparticipant inquiry. Whatever classificatory schemas we use in our efforts to order the diversity of psychoanalytic praxis, and however complex our theorizing and metatheorizing becomes, the basic facts of the clinical psychoanalytic situation remain invariant. All theories of psychoanalytic therapy represent differing conceptual perspectives on the inevitably coparticipatory nature of the analytic process. The psychoanalytic encounter, like all human relatedness, inherently defines or involves an intersubjective or coparticipant experience. This fundamental property of the analytic inquiry encompasses two intertwined clinical dimensions: (1) dyadic interactivity and reactivity, and (2) psychic subjectivity, in both (a) immediate experience and (b) reflective structuring of meaning.

The psychoanalytic process is, in other words, essentially three-dimensional in nature—at once relational, narrational, and experiential. Invariably and irreducibly, each and every analytic inquiry, though individually and uniquely patterned, is built out of these interpenetrating elements: a human relationship between two people; an effort to form (discover, uncover, construct, or deconstruct) a personally meaningful narrative or interpretation of one's life; and a lived experience of that process and relationship. These dimensions define the analytic process in both microscopic and macroscopic ways. Any concrete moment, specific analytic process or dynamic (psychic action, interaction, fantasy, etc.) or part of a session is complexly woven from interpersonal, interpretive, and experiential analytic strands.

Similarly, on a macroscopic level, these dimensions may be seen as phases of the overall process of any particular psychoanalysis. In a sense, all technical controversies in clinical psychoanalysis derive fundamentally from differing perspectives on these analytic dimensions and ultimately from one's concept of analytic participation or coparticipation.

Contemporary psychoanalytic praxis, as noted earlier, seems to draw from three broad clinical perspectives or models of inquiry: the impersonal *nonparticipant mirror*, the interpersonal *participant-observer*, and the personal *coparticipant inquiry*.

These clinical models or paradigms differ fundamentally in their under-standing of the three essential analytic dimensions, and they represent sig-nificantly different conceptions of psychoanalytic data, technique, and process; in other words, they are positioned quite differently on the dual clinical axes of dyadic interactivity and psychic subjectivity. And, of course, they represent different perspectives on the nature of analytic par-ticipation. The various traditionally defined analytic schools have bor-rowed from all three models, though some schools lean more heavily on one or another model to guide their understanding of analytic inquiry.

The impersonally oriented *nonparticipant mirror* paradigm encom-passes the orthodox analytic theory of inquiry whose guiding metaphor of the analysis is that of the nonparticipant mirror or psychic surgeon who reflects and interpretively operates on the transferential biopsychic fan-tasies of the individual patient. This is the model of inquiry prescribed by Freud and practiced most purely by the American neoclassicists of the 1950s. Even today, it remains the most widely held view of what is proper psychoanalysis.

The interpersonally focused *participant-observer* paradigm, in con-trast, focuses on the social mind, the interpsyche, as it arises from the social field; the interpretive and experiential interplay of self and other within the interpersonal analytic matrix forms both analytic data and therapeutic action. This model of inquiry informs the clinical approach of a wide range of analysts who practice some variant of participant-obser-vation, however widely they may differ from one another in other respects. This paradigm covers the heterogeneous span of British object-relations theory, the American school of interpersonal psychoanalysis, and Kohutian self-psychology, as well as some contemporary Freudians.

The deeply personal clinical model of *coparticipant inquiry*, histori-cally rooted in the clinical ideas and experiments of Sandor Ferenczi, is based on the interpersonally oriented participant-observer paradigm but has a more personal and intersubjective focus. In this model of praxis, analyst and patient are seen as forming a coparticipatory and coordinate inquiry into both their interpersonal relatedness and their uniquely indi-vidual experience. The coparticipant model emphasizes the importance of real factors in transference and countertransference experience as well as the curative role of the personal relationship. This model of inquiry, which also bears an existential influence, significantly informs (often uncon-sciously) the work of a number of contemporary analysts and is becom-ing increasingly influential in its effect on analytic practice.

Each of the three paradigms I posit here has or has had some influence on the traditionally defined psychoanalytic schools, even if only mini-mally in some instances. Each school has found the logic of one or another paradigm, its particular premises and emphases, more compelling or compatible than those of the other paradigms. The emergence of these major paradigms represents focal attempts to comprehend the fundamental nature of the analytic encounter and an effort to find the approach that is clinically most fruitful for the psychoanalytic situation. Each of these paradigms also arose in response to other factors—intellectual and philosophical trends, social currents, previous paradigmatic beliefs, emerging clinical problems (tied to previous paradigmatic limitations), new trends in psychopathology and in its diagnosis, clinical discoveries, trends in psychoanalytic sensibility, and the general spirit of the times.

The different paradigms have generally followed a historical path, from the classical conception of the analyst as nonparticipant blank screen to the interpersonal participant-observer to the coparticipant inquirer. All the paradigms have been influential since the early days of psychoanalytic therapy, but each one came to dominate psychoanalytic praxis in certain historical periods.

My classificatory schema of clinical paradigms or models, like all such efforts at classification, is inevitably Procrustean, despite its heuristic merit. It simplifies and clarifies the complex, bewildering plethora of analytic problems and practices, but it misses the individuality and particularity of each coparticipant psychoanalytic situation.

A fundamental feature of the psychoanalytic encounter is its coparticipant nature, expressed clinically in interactivity and experienced subjectivity. The three psychoanalytic paradigms I posit offer different ways of seeing the nature of the coparticipatory analytic encounter and its constituent psychic subjectivity and dyadic interactivity. The different paradigms guide analysts' conceptions of the nature and sanctioned or proper use of their analytic coparticipation, shaping their understanding of their integration with their patients. All questions, issues, and personal rules of analytic conduct spring ultimately from one's concept of his or her participation in inquiry—from one's ideas about the meaning, value, and impact of his or her analytic coparticipation.

Coparticipation refers to both the intrapsychic and the interpsychic, to the inner psychological world and the outer material world, and to their dynamic and often reciprocal relationship. Analytic coparticipation does not mean only what is visible in behavior, but it refers also to what is felt and thought, to the processes of the mind, as in listening, thinking, judging, evaluating, feeling, wanting, remembering, etc.

The psychoanalytic relationship is, without exception, a special instance of human coparticipation. All questions of technique and process derive fundamentally from one's concept of his or her coparticipant engagement with his or her patient. The three paradigms of analytic participation cut across traditional theoretical lines. Most analysts who practice some form of coparticipant inquiry identify themselves in terms of their metapsychological affiliations or schools, such as interpersonal, self-psychological, Freudian, Jungian, Kleinian, etc., rather than in terms of the model of praxis that guides or informs their way of working.

My aim here is not to give the definitive word on coparticipant inquiry; rather, I want to draw attention to emerging coparticipant trends in psychoanalytic praxis that push us to the farther edges of accepted analytic investigation. This book is an exploration of an emerging unique psychoanalytic paradigm that promises an innovative approach to the analytic task. In my exploration of the coparticipant themes and concepts that arise in the study of such psychoanalytic phenomena as the therapeutic dialectics of the multidimensional self, the dynamics and therapeutics of narcissistic processes, the "living through" process, the "analytic working space," and the therapeutic implications of "openness to singularity," I will touch upon the central controversies in clinical psychoanalysis. This includes a discussion of questions such as: What defines the most effective approach to transference analysis? What is the role of extratransference inquiry? What are the promises and perils of countertransference analysis? What is the analytic role of regression? How do analysts listen? What is the role of dream analysis? What is the nature of therapeutic action in psychoanalysis?

These questions represent some of the major questions and controversies that divide contemporary analysts who draw from different paradigms or models of inquiry. In sum, the clinical controversies that characterize contemporary psychoanalytic praxis derive from different conceptions of the coparticipant psychoanalytic situation and its constituent processes of dyadic interactivity and psychic subjectivity. An analyst's position on these clinical axes determines his or her theoretical understanding of psychoanalysis and the analyst's role in it as well as the details of his or her praxis and its therapeutic potential.

PART ONE

COPARTICIPATION

CHAPTER 1

Coparticipation and Coparticipant Inquiry

COPARTICIPATION

All psychoanalyses, however symbolized or structured, are coparticipatory integrations. The psychoanalytic situation always involves two unique personalities, entwined in double-helix fashion, continuously transferring experience, resisting influence, suffering anxiety, and analyzing themselves and each other. As the prefix *co*, meaning "with," "joint," "mutual," "in conjunction," suggests, analyst and patient are inevitably *coparticipants*—interrelated within an interpersonal field of their making, inextricably involved in a continuous series of reciprocal interactions.

Both analyst and patient bring their conscious and unconscious motives, wishes, and ideals—their personal strivings and stirrings, interpersonal insecurities, defensive striving, and relational yearnings—to their shared relationship. Consequently, they will interact around these psychic realities for as long as they remain in relationship with one another.

Fundamentally, psychoanalysis is a human encounter—a meeting of two beings or two minds (Aron 1996) in all their unique individuality. The coparticipants each bring to their shared relationship their unique expectations, desires, and abilities as well as their imagination, curiosity, and courage.

Coparticipation is a psychoanalytic given, whether one grasps this clinical fact and builds one's inquiry upon it, or repudiates it and limits its vital potential for analytic inquiry. From the beginning, analysts have recognized the clinical reality that they and their patients actively participate with one another throughout an analysis. This simple fact, however, has been understood and treated in widely different ways, and in some instances its central role in coparticipant experience has even been denied. These differences reflect how analysts of different schools have variously conceptualized—decided how to think "correctly"—the coparticipant nature of the psychoanalytic situation and the two-person psychology of its dyadic integration. Historically, within classical psychoanalysis conceptions of the analytic process, from those of Freud (1912, 1913, 1915) through those of Menninger (1958), Greenson (1967), and Brenner (1976), have tended to limit the role of patients as true copartners, assigning them a more restricted psychoanalytic role. Nevertheless, many theorists, including Freud, practiced more liberally, freely, and personally than what they put forth in their theories of treatment; in some instances, they disregarded in practice the technique they formally prescribed for others. However, some analysts searched openly for their own answers. Psychoanalytic pioneers of an independent spirit, such as Franz Alexander, Otto Rank, and most notably Sandor Ferenczi tried to treat patients in more fully coparticipant terms. Nevertheless, most classical analysts hewed to the restrictive limits of acceptable Freudian orthodoxy, some more rigidly so than others.

One can certainly see the merits of such technical aims as analytic objectivity, impartiality, tact, judicious reserve, and authoritative knowledge. It was, in part, to facilitate the use of such clinical techniques or attitudes that Freud and his successors developed the impersonal technique of orthodox psychoanalysis. Freud had another reason for a canon of impersonal techniques and limited coparticipation. He feared that psychoanalysis, with its deeply personal and subjective nature, was subject to the criticism of achieving therapeutic results by virtue of suggestion (i.e., relational influence), that in essence psychoanalysis was simply a form of interpersonal hypnosis. Freud feared that psychoanalysis would be considered unscientific, and he understandably wished to develop it in terms of the science of his day. So he called for purity in the analytic situation.

This meant an emphasis on the analyst's neutrality, anonymity, and interpretive authority and called for the patient's abstinence, literal or metaphoric. In short, Freud argued for a highly circumscribed form of the coparticipant psychoanalytic relationship. The analytic doctor, as interpretive surgeon, knowing what was best, would operate upon the resistant patient. So the patient got the silent treatment, in more ways than one.

This restrictive technique, however, also represented what Freud himself needed or thought he needed in order to work with patients, and his followers adopted the same method. However, as noted earlier, those who were free to recognize the clinical implications of analytic coparticipation and who possessed the personal freedom and desire to work with their patients in a more coparticipant manner did so. In the process they found ways to resolve their dilemmas of personal versus institutional or theoretical loyalty, the question of whether to be true to their own natural way of working or to adhere to the teachings of the analytic canon, the prescribed path.

The British school of object relations opened the door to a more coparticipatory view of the analytic hour, attending, for example, to the clinical study of the mutual influences and complex intersubjective transactions that inevitably occur between patient and analyst, each contributing to the shaping of the other's clinical experience. However, analytic participation still remained relatively circumscribed. The authoritarian mirror analyst had become the authoritarian mirroring analyst, the analytic good parent who knew best what the patient needed. The analyst, though no longer silent, detached, or rigid, was still the authority who had the final word. Thus, object relations theory began to focus on the critical interplay of transference and countertransference experience, the vast, complex, and constantly changing coparticipatory processes that characterize all analytic situations. However, there was no corresponding shift toward a comprehensive, bidirectional, and radical coparticipatory way of working. Nevertheless, this analytic approach, though often practiced in orthodox, authoritarian ways, represents a move toward a more coparticipatory inquiry.

The work of Kohut and post-Kohutian analysts, too, has recognized the interactive or transactive—i.e., intersubjective—nature of each person's relatedness and found that psychoanalytic relatedness in the clinical situation was profound and pervasive, that patient and analyst essentially were each a coparticipant. But again, technique and inquiry remained circumscribed and fairly traditional. Kohut proposed a metapsychology that was vastly different from Freud's and replaced or supplemented Freud's libido theory with a theory of an interpersonal self that emphasized the primacy of reflected interpersonal appraisals and influences in psychic development and functioning. Nevertheless, Kohut (1971, 1977, 1984) failed to extend or alter or even enlarge neoclassical clinical thinking. His technique, as he asserted, was the same as Freud's. Though Kohut emphasized the clinical primacy of a radically empathic listening stance and though he strove, in Rogerian (cf. Rogers 1951) spirit, to follow the patient's needs for interpersonal security or self-other (what Kohut termed "self-object") experience, this same patient was not admitted to the analytic hour as a full copartner or coparticipant inquirer, at least not in terms of his or her analytic capacities. Rather, the patient was defined implicitly as the analytic child, forlorn and forsaken, or starry-eyed and symbiotic, but not a copartner. In this sense, Kohut (whom I will return to in my discussion of the self in chapters 4 and 5), vitiates the promise, based upon the study of the intersubjective nature of the psychoanalytic field of experience and its natural influences, of conceptualizing analytic work as a coparticipatory process.

The clinical approaches of Kohut and the English object relationists strongly resemble the analytic perspective of the seminal American interpersonalist Harry Stack Sullivan for whom the analyst is, or should be, an expert in interpersonal relations. His expert was not of a family parent sort, but rather the expert interlocutor, the researcher who conducts a detailed inquiry into the patient's difficulties. It was Sullivan (1940, 1953) who first mapped the psychic dimension of interpersonal security or social adaptation that the object-relational analysts also emphasized in their clinical approaches. However, as already noted, this dimension comprised the study of the patient by the expert analyst, not a true study of *both* the patient and analyst by *both* the patient and analyst. Nevertheless, Sullivan saw clearly that the analyst is always involved in an interpersonal field—a dynamic system of reciprocal transactions that includes all who are part of it. The analyst, in Sullivan's (1953) view, was inevitably a *participant-observer*, a participant in and thus a part of what he or she studied. Sullivan's conceptions of the analyst as a participant-observer summarized and gave theoretical voice to the ideas and sensibilities of those analysts who could be said to have advocated or practiced some form of participant analytic inquiry.

Sullivan's participatory conceptions, radical for their time, were seminal and far-reaching. Nevertheless, they, too, had limitations and imposed restrictions on the living out of a full coparticipatory analysis. The analyst was *the* analyst and the patient was *the patient and nothing more*. The theory did not view analytic work as a coanalysis of both patient and analyst. Patient and analyst were simply not viewed as equals in analysis. Yet Sullivan's interpersonal contributions have played a major role in the development of coparticipant analytic inquiry. Today, many modern analysts, from a variety of theoretical perspectives and schools of thought, practice some form of coparticipant inquiry. In particular, contemporary interpersonal analysts developed more comprehensive versions of Sullivan's approach to the psychoanalytic situation. Recognition and appreciation of the coparticipatory nature of the analytic relationship has also marked recent clinical theorizing of some modern Freudians (see, for example, Jacobs 1991, 1998; Renik 1993, 2000). There also has been a burgeoning interest in coparticipatory concepts and practices, although often framed in other terms, among analysts who label themselves as "intersubjectivists," "relationists," or modern "object relationists" (see, for example, the work of Aron 1991, 2000; Bass 2001a,b, 2003; Stolorow, Atwood, and Brandchaft 1994).

This, in turn, has led to the formulation of various versions of coparticipant inquiry (though not put in this language), ranging from the relatively narrow to the comprehensive.[1] As will be discussed more fully in chapter

3, beyond a common repudiation of orthodox impersonal techniques, there is considerable diversity in the form of coparticipant inquiry practiced in these various relational clinical approaches.

The concept of coparticipation carries a dual meaning. It refers first of all to a universal characteristic of all analytic integrations (and all human relationships). Most simply stated, coparticipation refers to the inherently interactive and intersubjective, as well as intrasubjective, nature of the analytic relationship. Second, coparticipation refers to a particular form of clinical *inquiry*, which may be defined as one that takes into account the unique interpsychic and interactional nature of the analyst-patient relationship and addresses its implications for therapeutic procedure and process.

In modern psychoanalysis this form of inquiry is most closely approximated in the work of some contemporary analysts with an interpersonal and intersubjective orientation. Coparticipant inquiry is not associated with any one school of psychoanalysis, but it is most fully developed in the interpersonal school and, more recently, in post-Kohutian intersubjective psychoanalysis and other relational offshoots. Various forms of coparticipant inquiry characterize the psychoanalytic metaschool called relational theory. This metaschool includes social constructivist theory, intersubjectivity theory, self-psychology, various forms of object-relations psychology, some aspects of contemporary Freudian theory, and interpersonal psychoanalysis. Analysts of these various relational schools practice some form of coparticipant inquiry. Most of these contemporary analysts are relatively limited in their coparticipatory approach despite their relational metapsychologies and post-Cartesian epistemologies. The most comprehensive expression of coparticipant inquiry is the form practiced by those analysts who make up the "radical empiricist" wing of contemporary interpersonal psychoanalysis (see chapter 3 for a definition of radical empiricism).

Coparticipation *as a quality of relatedness* defines the interactive features of the interpersonal field that constitutes psychoanalysis (i.e., two unique selves in therapeutic interaction). Coparticipation *as a concept of inquiry*, derived from the coparticipatory nature of the analytic situation and process, represents a therapeutic sensibility and clinical philosophy, a way of living psychoanalysis, rather than a defined set of techniques, clinical strategies, or rules of praxis.

Coparticipation, as a description of the fundamental intersubjective nature of all psychoanalytic relationships, is not a new phenomenon—interaction is a fundamental fact and facet of all psychoanalyses. What is new is the growing recognition of the clinical promise of coparticipant inquiry as a new clinical paradigm. While coparticipant inquiry, recognizing the coparticipant nature of the psychoanalytic situation, is predominantly a modern movement in psychoanalytic practice, its roots reach back to the early history of psychoanalysis and the radical clinical experiments of Sandor Ferenczi.

One may ask: why use the term "coparticipation" instead of simply using the better known term "participation." I use the word coparticipation to emphasize the intrinsic mutuality, motivational reciprocity, psychic symmetry, coequality of analytic authority, and participatory bidirectionality of the analytic relationship, whether or not one or both coparticipants choose to deny or ignore these clinical possibilities and proceed to work on some basis that fails to attend to this clinical reality.

In the psychoanalytic situation, coparticipant processes flow continuously, even if denied or restricted by the analyst's metapsychological, clinical, or personal prejudices and preferences. Any psychoanalytic dyad or member of that dyad, out of personal reserve, personal inclination, obsessional need for control, or other pertinent reasons, may proscribe inquiry into particular aspects of their coparticipant functioning and experience. There is in such instances an ongoing *coparticipant process* but not a full *coparticipant inquiry* into that process. Nevertheless, in the coparticipant experience formed by the two copartners, as noted earlier, each inevitably brings all of himself or herself into the analytic situation, whether or not this is recognized and worked with. *In other words, all analyses are coparticipant processes, but not all are coparticipant inquiries.*

Coparticipant inquiry, the therapeutic use of coparticipant principles, does not require any particular metapsychology, nor does it represent a particular school of psychoanalysis. However, it usually finds a warmer welcome among modern interpersonalists or those contemporary analysts who are working relationally or intersubjectively. In its salient features coparticipant inquiry does not, as many historical new forms of psychoanalytic treatment do, represent the creation or discovery of a new metapsychology from which a new technique or psychoanalytic method is then derived. Coparticipation does not derive from a metapsychology. Born in clinical practice and therapeutically primary, coparticipant inquiry evolves instead from an awareness of the specific limitations of other, prior, forms of clinical inquiry.

How, then, do we define this new psychoanalytic approach? What features define this way of working and thinking? How does coparticipant inquiry differ from, for example, orthodox Freudian treatment conceptions or those of relational analysis? Let's turn to a consideration of such questions.

COPARTICIPANT INQUIRY

Coparticipant inquiry is premised on the awareness of the intersubjective nature of the clinical situation and the commitment to working with its therapeutic potentialities. What distinguishes coparticipant inquiry is not a specific set of prescribed techniques nor a specific technical canon. Coparticipatory practice represents, instead, a clinical attitude or approach, a way of working and of being with the patient, that leads spontaneously to clinical actions consistent with the core principles of coparticipant inquiry (reviewed in chapter 2). Coparticipant inquiry does not call for *the* one right way to do analytic work; there is only the question of whether one's work is true to the clinical reality of his or her coparticipant experience.

Whether they are aware of it or not, even the most conservative analysts, in varying degrees and in various ways, practice some principles of coparticipant inquiry (that is, an inquiry that takes cognizance of the complex two-way coparticipant nature of the psychoanalytic situation). However, few practice it fully or consistently.

Analysts of the different psychoanalytic schools view the coparticipatory nature of the analytic situation in dramatically different terms; some repudiate this view of the analytic process while others embrace this clinical perspective and its radical clinical implications. How is this clinical modality best defined? Coparticipant psychoanalytic inquiry, when practiced consistently, is characterized by seven interrelated features or principles; individually and jointly, these principles carry a number of clinical implications and therapeutic consequences:

1. The analytic situation is seen as an interpersonal field within which patients and analysts create a shared field of experience. The coparticipants, patient and analyst, bring the totality of their individual psychic resources and life experiences to their interactive union. Together they forge a dyadic encounter unique to them. In short, the coparticipant psychoanalytic situation involves two people, each influencing the other, jointly shaping the unique course and nature of their relationship.

2. Analytic relatedness is seen as a working dialectic between interpersonal processes (intersubjectivity) and personal processes (unique individuality)—in other words, between social adaptiveness and individual self-expression. This brings to psychoanalytic practice a concept of a *personal*, nonrelational, self in dynamic relation to an *interpersonal* self. With the concept of personal "I" processes, of unique individuality and capability, such concepts as will, choice, self-determination, and agency come into analytic play. Moreover, the range of analytic metapsychologies expands to include personal fulfillment, or self-actualization, as a central dynamic.

3. Analysts and patients are treated as analytic equals, *coanalysts*. Both analyst and patient are seen as continuously involved (to the best of their ability and desire) in the analysis of their transferential, resistant,

and anxious coparticipation with each other. Thus, patients are actively encouraged to take a proactive role as analytic copartners.

4. Patients' personal and interpersonal *responsiveness, responsibility, and resourcefulness* are recognized and emphasized. Patients and analysts alike are seen as both open to interpersonal influence and as simultaneously self-determining.

5. *Metapsychological (interpretive) and methodological (technical)* pluralism is emphasized. A radical individuation of interpretive myth and metaphor and of analytic method is encouraged.

6. A *technically bold, self-expressive, and spontaneous inquiry* is supported.

7. The therapeutic importance of *immediate experience* is emphasized as opposed to the traditional focus on the curative primacy of formulative interpretation.

These characteristics or features of coparticipant inquiry comprise a view of the analyst's expertise as residing not in his or her "expert" knowledge of metapsychologically derived psychodynamics or institutionally determined proper technique but rather in his or her skills and capacities for facilitating and participating in an alive, creative, and imaginative inquiry.

The notion of the analyst as an expert who knows (or can know) the answers to the patient's neurotic dilemmas implies that the analyst is omnipotent. In a coparticipant inquiry, the analyst is not required to be the superior participant who knows best, the arbiter of analytic reality and proper method. Instead, the analyst's task is to encourage, facilitate, and to some extent guide the patient's therapeutic developmental process—to help the patient realize his or her own psychic resources and his or her own directions, preferences, intuitions, and wisdom. In other words, the analyst helps the patient to find his or her own answers, which previously had been anxiously avoided. Coparticipant analysts foster their patients' growth as catalytic agents, helping them develop independent functions previously undeveloped. Though analysts may not know best, it is assumed that they have developed some wisdom about life and the human condition that may prove helpful to the patients they work with. In coparticipant therapy the obverse also applies; that is, the patient may provide insights into the analyst's difficulties and, accordingly, may contribute to his or her participatory partner's development. Ideally, coparticipant inquiry facilitates or creates the analytic conditions or relational atmosphere that prompts the therapeutic emergence of both *regressive* and *progressive* aspects of the patient's psychic functioning. The analyst creates the personal freedom for both regressive and progressive elements of his or her own psychic being to emerge as appropriate for therapeutic understanding by both coparticipants.

The seven features schematically outlined here and discussed in greater detail in chapter 2 define the specific nature of coparticipant psychoanalytic inquiry when practiced comprehensively. The therapeutic use of any one aspect of this approach does not mark an analyst as a practitioner of coparticipant analysis, which requires the consistent application of all seven principles. Some analysts only approximate coparticipant analysis, often practicing it in attenuated form. Yet, some form of coparticipant inquiry, however limited, is practiced in all schools of psychoanalysis, certainly by analysts belonging to the relational metafamily of psychoanalysis. The practice of coparticipant inquiry cuts across traditional theoretical boundaries, for, as noted earlier, it is not associated exclusively with any one school of analytic thought or practice. In fact, analysts who practice some form of coparticipant inquiry have not, until the recent work of Benjamin Wolstein and other modern interpersonalists, identified themselves as such because they did not think of themselves as belonging to a coparticipant school or even as practicing according to coparticipant principles.

Coparticipant inquiry represents a clinical paradigm, a perspective, as it were, on psychoanalytic therapy. Most psychoanalysts identify with their chosen school, which is usually defined in terms of its predominant metapsychology or theory of human psychology. It is interesting that analytic clinicians have traditionally identified with one or another prevailing metapsychology, rather than with a particular clinical orientation that may cut across metapsychological or school lines (although metapsychological affiliations often result in particular choices of clinical orientation).

THREE PSYCHOANALYTIC PARADIGMS

Although most analysts at times use coparticipatory concepts of inquiry, they mainly work according to a different set of therapeutic concepts. The history of psychoanalytic praxis suggests that there have been three paradigms of analytic participation or praxis and thus three fundamentally different ways of working: nonparticipant observation, participant-observation, and coparticipant inquiry.

Nonparticipant Observation

Briefly, the nonparticipant model of praxis, what Wolstein (1959, 1977a) called the mirror-observational model, refers to the neoclassical, orthodox model of psychoanalytic practice in which the analyst is seen as the interpretive surgeon who in an "objective," detached manner observes and operates on the neurotic, dysfunctional intrapsychic or inner fantasy life of the similarly distanced patient. In this way of working, the analyst is the interpretive authority, the sole arbiter of clinical reality. Thus, this analytic modal-

ity, marked by a profound asymmetry, requires and values analytic impersonality (i.e., "blank screen")—in some instances, to the point of absurdity.
This approach minimizes the patient's therapeutic role and contributions. It
tends to discount the patient's desires to participate more actively. The nonparticipant analyst strives for an analytic anonymity and neutrality that is
impossible to achieve. Self-disclosure in this setting is also necessarily limited.

This model of therapy, limited as it is, still represents for many analysts the model of proper psychoanalytic technique. It often plays a significant role in the therapeutic superegos of even those analysts who
largely repudiate this view of analytic work. Of course, even among
those most influenced by this approach there are significant individual
variations in clinical temperament, sensibility, and in the adoption of the
principles of nonparticipant analysis and their application.

Despite its obvious flaws and untenable premises (for example, that the
analyst can be a "blank screen," a pristine mirror, and knows what is best
and what is real), this clinical model attempts to realize, as far as it is possible, analytic objectivity, therapeutic balance, care in inquiry, respect for
the patients' need for psychological space to connect with their processes,
and judicious self-revelation—that is, analysts working with this approach
take care not to intrude or impinge unnecessarily upon the patient.

Historically, this clinical model was developed, in part, to assure the scientific status of psychoanalytic therapy, to buttress the new discipline
against objections that analysis was "wild," ill informed, and not under
rational control. Freud was particularly concerned that the therapeutic
results of psychoanalytic treatment not be dismissed as unscientific, due to
"suggestion" or personal influence. Hence the imperative to pattern psychoanalytic therapy and the patient-analyst relationship on the methodology of
the so-called hard physical sciences of the day. Freud and his followers were
guided by the principle that events are best studied in pure isolation, and
they strove to achieve a purified rather than participatory analytic field.

In recent years, many practitioners who adhere to this model of analytic
participation (or nonparticipation) have been influenced by the tenets of
the *participant-observer model* of psychoanalytic praxis and have softened
previous rigidly held, authoritarian ideas about psychoanalytic therapy.

Participant-Observation

The *participant-observer* clinical paradigm amounts to a revolution in psychoanalytic technique and clinical sensibility. This model of treatment
repudiates the impersonal technique of the nonparticipant model and
found its earliest expression in the interpersonal relational conceptions of
Harry Stack Sullivan who coined the term participant-observer to describe
the inevitable participatory nature of the analyst's work. The coparticipa-

tory sensibility of the American school of interpersonal relations also found expression in the cognate concepts of the early British object-relations approaches of Melanie Klein, D. W. Winnicott, and R. D. W. Fairbairn, among others. The participant-observation paradigm emphasizes the interactive and intersubjective nature—what some call a two-person psychology—of the analytic process. It now characterizes the work of a heterogeneous group of American interpersonalists, Kohutian self-psychologists, contemporary Freudians, ego-psychologists, and British object-relationists that has been gathered under the metatheoretical umbrella of the "relational" family of psychoanalysis. The emphasis on the mutual influence of patient and analyst—the analytic situation as an interpersonal field—is the hallmark that divides the participant-observer paradigm from the earlier orthodox, nonparticipant paradigm.

The coparticipant model has evolved out of the participant-observer model. For Sullivan, as for many analysts of other relational schools, participant observation—unlike coparticipant inquiry—represents a one-way view of the analytic process: there is only one analyst, the expert participant-observer. The analyst is the expert in interpersonal relations who conducts the therapeutic inquiry and defines both analytic methodology and analytic metapsychology. Thus, participant-observation offers no radical individuation of methodology or metapsychology nor any acceptance of the therapeutic benefits of working directly with the uniquely individual aspects of the patient's or the analyst's personality. This tends to be true of the work of other analysts of a broadly relational orientation. For example, Kohut (1971, 1977) and Winnicott (1958, 1965) viewed interpersonal or object-relational treatment in one-way relational terms and saw the analyst as mirroring self-object or as holding mother. In participant-observation the analyst and patient are seen in a superordinate-subordinate hierarchical relationship with each other.

Thus, although the participant-observer model of praxis differs from the nonparticipatory model in placing the analyst squarely within the interpersonal field of analysis, it nevertheless remains authoritarian—the analyst still knows best. Full recognition of the coparticipatory status of the patient is denied, which limits the study of the transference-countertransference relationship and of the personal, nontransferential relationship (see chapter 8). Participant-observers are not mythically neutral mirrors, but neither are they what they could be: full coparticipants, experiencing, interpreting, observing, and inquiring jointly.

Coparticipant Inquiry

The participant-observer paradigm has gradually evolved into the *coparticipatory model* of psychoanalytic practice. As previously noted, this has happened particularly in the work of analysts of the American interpersonalist school, especially Benjamin Wolstein and Edgar Levenson. Wolstein (1959, 1997) observed that the analyst is not only a participant-observer but equally and simultaneously also an observed-participant. In short, a *co*participant. In a seminal series of papers, Wolstein (1977a,b, 1981a,b, 1983a,b, 1988), who coined the term *coparticipant inquiry*, articulated the therapeutic potential and possibilities of mutual analysis and mutual analytic engagement of the uniquely individual aspects of patients and analysts. In a very different, but equally original, set of studies, Levenson (1972, 1983, 1991) pointed to the coparticipatory transformation of the analyst by the patient in inevitable analytic reenactments of early traumas. Levenson's ideas anticipated by twenty-five years the current coparticipant study of analytic enactments and the co-created patterning of transference-countertransference relatedness by analysts who come from a nonparticipant tradition.

The classificatory schema presented here briefly, like all classificatory efforts, is inevitably Procrustean. Analysts select from all three paradigms. Moreover, there are overlapping features in the practices associated with the different modes of praxis. Nevertheless, this typology holds true as a schematic for how analysts clinically set themselves apart from each other.

Many analysts (and patients), as just noted, incorporate elements or aspects of coparticipant inquiry in their predominantly noncoparticipatory methodology. The practice of coparticipant inquiry ranges from minimal use of coparticipant principles to extensive and even extremist uses of such concepts. Each analyst characteristically tends to work somewhere along that continuum, which may vary with changes in the nature of analytic themes (i.e., the problem addressed), the particular patient involved, the current state of the analysis, the period or phase of the work, and various other analytic contingencies.

For various complex cultural, political, or clinical reasons, each of the different paradigms have been found to be influential and useful at different periods in the history of psychoanalysis. The future of psychoanalytic praxis, however, belongs to the evolving and emergent paradigm of coparticipant inquiry, with its emphasis on the analyst's deep personal involvement in the shared experiential therapeutic field.

In chapter 3 I will describe in greater detail the evolution of coparticipant inquiry in clinical psychoanalysis. First, however, let's take a closer look at the defining features or core principles of this form of coparticipation.

CHAPTER 2

Core Principles of
Coparticipant Inquiry

Coparticipant inquiry is defined by seven interrelated clinical features; when practiced consistently, they distinguish this form of analytic inquiry from all others. As noted in chapter 1, these core principles are the following:

1. An understanding of the psychoanalytic situation as an interpersonal and intersubjective field of experience. This constitutes the analytic importance of the *relational* and *interpersonal* dimensions of the self.

2. A recognition of and emphasis on the psychoanalytic importance of unique individuality, including the capacity for will, choice, and proactive motivation. This constitutes the clinical influence of the *personal* dimension of the self.

3. A view of the patient as an analytic copartner to the full extent of his or her ability.

4. An emphasis on both patients' and analysts' personal responsibility and interpersonal responsivity.

5. A radical individuation of metapsychologies and methodology. Every analysis is seen as a unique event, both personally and interpersonally.

6. A radical view of the psychoanalytic process which includes freedom of self-expression and self-disclosure, active use of countertransference experience, an informal clinical atmosphere, and a repudiation of neutrality and anonymity on the part of the analyst.

7. An appreciation of the importance of immediate experience in psychoanalytic exploration and new relational experience in therapeutic cure.

These seven principles thus constitute coparticipant inquiry. Taken as a whole and practiced comprehensively, they define a distinctive form of inquiry that incorporates concepts from other forms of analytic inquiry (e.g., participant-observation) but yet remains unique in itself. Let's now take a closer look at these core principles of coparticipant inquiry; we'll begin with an examination of the relation of coparticipation to field theory.

THE INTERPERSONAL FIELD

The concept of the psychoanalytic situation as an interpersonal and intersubjective field is central to coparticipant theory. Coparticipant inquiry is premised on a field concept of the analytic relationship. Patients and analysts are seen as interactively creating a therapeutic relationship marked by psychic symmetry, mutual influence, and motivational reciprocity. In this shared *experiential field*, unique to its coparticipant creators, patients and analysts alike bring to their relationship their psychic being and becoming—rational and irrational, conscious and unconscious—and they live these out in the dynamic interplay of their respective transferences and countertransferences, self-protecting resistances and counterresistances, confusing anxieties and counteranxieties, and maturing and centering relatedness. In their shared communicative and affective fields of experience, patient and analyst, in continuous, intersecting relation to one another, observe, explore, analyze, and work through mutual problems and possibilities in living.

Psychological field theory, borrowed originally from the late nineteenth-century physics of Faraday, Maxwell, Herz, and other field theorists, first found psychological expression in the early twentieth century field-theoretical perceptual studies of the Gestalt school of Wertheimer, Koffka, Kohler, and, later, in the personality studies of Kurt Lewin. In fact, field theory is implicit in much of contemporary thinking on psychoanalytic therapy and historically emerged in the seminal interpersonal psychoanalytic concepts of Harry Stack Sullivan. Contemporary interpersonalists who practice a more radical form of coparticipant inquiry consider transference an unavoidable part of a complex transference-countertransference matrix. Transference and countertransference are thus viewed as reciprocal, co-created, and interpenetrating field processes.

Every patient-analyst relationship is seen to represent a uniquely configured dyad, in which patient and analyst are constantly and mutually influencing one another. Thus, in coparticipant inquiry *both the analyst's and the patient's personalities are studied, by both patient and analyst.* Transference and countertransference are seen as mutually formed experiences created by both analytic coparticipants, rather than as exclusively endogenous expressions of either coparticipant's closed intrapsychic world. In other words, transference invariably shapes, and reveals itself, in the analyst's countertransference; conversely, the analyst's countertransference partly shapes, and reveals itself, in the patient's transference. Transference and countertransference thus represent an integral of self and situation: variable amalgams of the unconscious experience of both patient and analyst. A patient's transference hostility, for example, shapes itself to conform to the analyst's unconscious vulnerabilities. This same hostility would be expressed differently with different analysts, unconsciously tailored to fit the particular analyst's personality. In turn, different analysts would react differently, responding with various irrational and rational reactions, ranging from angry retaliation to masochistic submission to selective inattention or insightful clarity and compassion. The analysts's reaction in turn prompts different counterreactions from the patient, these then in turn prompt reactions from the analyst and so on in ever expanding, recursive complexity. Hence, from a coparticipant perspective, every analytic dyad is seen as generating its own unique transference-countertransference matrix of action and experience.

A central clinical implication of this conception of transference and countertransference is that understanding the patient's personality inevitably involves an understanding of the analyst's personality and vice-versa. Transference and countertransference analysis become integral aspects of one another. In this sense, transference and countertransference are indivisible interpersonal processes, reciprocal poles of a continuum of unconscious experience. Since countertransference contributes to the shaping and clinical unfolding of transference, its analysis by both patient and analyst is pertinent to the analysis of transference. Coparticipant analysts focus on both the patient's and their own experience of their analytic relatedness and, radically enough, invite their patient to do the same.

From this coparticipant viewpoint, monadic and noninteractive approaches to transference, even if they are relational in their interpretive metaphors, limit and distort analysts' understanding of their patients and themselves. For example, if a patient's transference experience, say, of curiosity about the analyst, is seen only as expression of some endogenous dynamic, such as primal sexuality, hostility, or infantile dependence, then other possible unconscious motivations, such as loving care, fearful ingratiation, or compassionate helpfulness, that are interactionally linked to the analyst's countertransference (e.g., his or her loneliness, exhibitionism, or desire for treatment) may be overlooked and the truer, more complex interactional meaning of the patient's transference may go unrecognized.

In sum, transference and countertransference, like resistance and counterresistance, and anxiety and counteranxiety, are generated in coparticipation: they are inevitable field processes, reciprocal poles of a complex, interactive experiential field. Consideration of either process always involves a consideration of its reciprocal counterpart. Coparticipant analysts view transference and countertransference as inextricably interrelated processes born out of the joint interaction between themselves and their patients. Accordingly, transference and countertransference form indivisible parts of a continuum of relatedness and experience. Therapeutically, their interactive nature and function are best understood by a thoroughgoing and uncompromising coparticipant inquiry.

The coparticipant view of transference and countertransference as field processes points to the general significance of context or surround in the assignment of meaning. Context is defined in manifold ways in coparticipant psychoanalytic inquiry. Any psychic act of the individual patient—a feeling state, an attitude, a pattern of behavior—may be seen in any or all of the following contexts: the patient's personal and interpersonal history; his or her personality features; the patient's biology; the contemporary or "here and now" interpersonal context; the pattern of previous sessions; the psychic reverberations and themes of the immediately preceding session; the anticipated next one; the pattern of parallel events outside analysis; and the cultural and historical values and prevailing belief systems in which this all happens. What is considered contextually relevant in any situation is, of course, itself contextually determined. The analyst's own situatedness—his or her theoretical convictions, therapeutic values, interpersonal anxieties, personal maturity—will figure into his or her conscious or unconscious choice of contextual lens. This lens may be wider or narrower and more or less variable or fixed.

A caveat is in order here: emphasizing the psychoanalytic field and contextual analysis can lead to an excessive focus on the social or interpersonal environment and to a relative neglect of the individual and the intrapsychic. The field perspective, though clinically invaluable, runs the risk of reducing the uniqueness of the individual to his or her relational participation. The emphasis on contextual meaning, which characterizes the psychological field concepts of such personality theorists as Kurt Lewin, Andras Angyal, and Gardner Murphy and defines the psychoanalytic field conceptions of Harry Stack Sullivan, reaches its most extreme expression in the field theories of contemporary family therapists and systems theorists. These approaches all focus on the determinative effects or contextual impact of social or psychological fields-of-force on their constituent coparticipants. A radical figure-ground methodology is emphasized: the part can *only* be understood by a study of the whole. From this one-sided perspective, separating figure from ground, part from whole, is to distort events and processes: individuals can only truly be known contextually.

Though a radically holistic analysis focusing on the systemic properties of interpersonal fields has therapeutic merit and takes into account that each analyst-patient field originates new interactive phenomena called by some "the analytic third," such an emphasis tends to reduce individuals to their field responsiveness, that is, to their interpersonal self. This limits, or even prohibits, a more comprehensive and complex understanding of the patient and his or her unique individuality. Prominent contemporary psychoanalytic concepts such as Klein's object-relational "projective identification," Levenson's interpersonal "transformed analyst," Sandler's relational "role-responsiveness," or Searles's supervisory "parallel process" because of their focus on *interpersonal influence* and *induced experience* carry the danger of seeing patients' or analysts' coparticipation as determined by their interpersonal field—that is, by the impact and counterimpact of the *other.* The analytic roles of agency, will, and self-determination are minimized, ignored, or dismissed.

Without an implicit or explicit concept of agency and individuality, a field theory must, inevitably, regard the patient and analyst as contextual victims—coercively transformed by the pressures of the surrounding field. With the atrophy of agency, influence becomes hypertrophied. Everything now becomes a matter of the other—of how you *make* me love, hate, fear, desire, disdain, and so on. Experience thus comes from without, rather than from within. Herein lies the danger of an overly interpersonalized or contextualized psychological study of another. Without a theory of a personal self and individuality, psychoanalytic field theory becomes overcontextualized, and the singularity of the patient and analyst gets lost in the field, as it were. At the same time, agency remains unaccounted for. A well-rounded coparticipant inquiry requires a concept of the "I," the person, as an active, striving being, a proactive initiator of experience and not simply a reactive receptor of influence. Of course, patient and analyst influence one another continually; if this were not so, there would be no therapy. Analyst and patient, however, are neither determined nor defined by their mutuality, only affected and influenced by it. If this were not so, we would be dealing with extreme psychological situationalism.[1]

A full account of a comprehensive coparticipant inquiry requires a notion of an active or proactive self. Coparticipant analysis, in its radical emphasis on patients' and analysts' active, expressive, and creative coparticipation and equal membership in the therapeutic experiential field, implies a concept of psychic centeredness and personal singularity.

Thus, we shall now turn to the second major feature of coparticipant inquiry—the dynamism of a personal self.

THE DYNAMICS OF THE PERSONAL SELF

Coparticipant inquiry is characterized by a unique dialectic. On the one hand, coparticipant inquiry represents a radical interpersonal concept of *co*partnered inquiry and readily appreciates the centrality of field dynamics, as expressed in mutual analysis. At the same time, coparticipant inquiry, especially in its more comprehensive forms, is characterized by a complementary appreciation of the unique individuality of the analytic participants (more accurately, *co*participants). This personal focus, when integrated in an ongoing dialectic between the radically social and the uniquely individual, distinguishes this form of psychoanalytic inquiry from others. This concept of coparticipant analysis, characterized by a dynamic relation of the personal and the interpersonal, can be diagrammed as shown in figure 2.1.

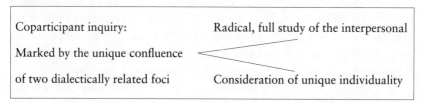

Coparticipant inquiry: Radical, full study of the interpersonal

Marked by the unique confluence

of two dialectically related foci   Consideration of unique individuality

Figure 2.1

Coparticipant psychoanalytic inquiry is premised on the dialectic of the dynamics of the personal self and the interpersonal self. In other words, coparticipant inquiry represents *both* a one-person and a two-person psychology, rather than just a one-person psychology (as in neoclassical Freudian orthodoxy) or a two-person psychology (as in most contemporary relational or interpersonal approaches).

Definitions seem in order. What do I mean by the "personal self"? And what is the "interpersonal self"? These concepts are described in detail in chapter 4, but I will briefly define and discuss them here in order to clarify their implications for coparticipant inquiry.

The dynamics of the *interpersonal self* refer to that domain of the self that arises out of a person's inherent need to socially adapt to the surrounding world of others. In Sullivan's theory, the self—what I call the "interpersonal self"—represents the sum of reflected appraisals by emotionally significant others. This representational patterning of "me" (or various "me's") is for Sullivan the inevitable product and eventual producer of social acculturation and adaptation. It reflects the universal human concern with social approval. This self formed out of the reflected opinion of others defines the same dimension of personality as Kohut's self or self-object relatedness—the human need for interpersonal security and freedom from the disorganizing effects of interpersonal anxiety (i.e., empathic failure). Though Sullivan and Kohut represent widely different clinical sensibilities, both theorists consider the interpersonal self and its (defensive) security operations and derivative character traits a central motivational dynamic.

In sharp contrast, the dynamics of the *personal self* refer to the individual strivings for self-realization and personal fulfillment, that is, the uniquely individual and personally authentic proactive aspects of a person's selfness. Thus, the personal self brings to the coparticipant inquiry's intersubjective, interpersonal field an individualistic, humanistic, and "existential" (in the sense of experiential) focus on emergent processes of will, choice, intention, self-determination, and the like. In coparticipant inquiry these are themes manifested in both spoken narrative and enacted transaction that the analyst and patient explicitly emphasize and attend to.

This has obvious clinical implications for coparticipant practice and for the ways in which patients are viewed. The patient is not seen simply as the suffering, transferential hurt child—the victim of unempathic circumstances—as many would have it. Instead, in coparticipant inquiry patients' interpersonal injuries (e.g., low self-esteem) and transferential fragility are recognized, noted, and worked with. At the same time, the patient is also seen as a resourceful and active, self-actualizing being who is striving to become himself or herself, as the psychologist Gordon Allport (1955) might put it. Explicit recognition of the psychic dimension of the personal self—what Wolstein refers to as the psychic center of the self—allows the analyst to look for and to facilitate the patient's awareness and articulation of his or her unique psychological powers and perspectives. This recognition of patients' (and analysts') personal selves, of their unique individuality and capability, is vital to the clinical establishment of the other characteristic features of coparticipant inquiry. When fully and authentically practiced, this leads to a more open, nonauthoritarian, and freer concept of inquiry.

The notion that each member of the analytic dyad (i.e., patient and analyst) possesses a singular selfness that actively seeks, however unconsciously, its own unique direction and development is integral to a radical, comprehensive coparticipant inquiry. It is the source that enables the patient (or analyst) to generate courage; face fears; bear grief, guilt, shame, and other dysphoric emotions; withstand therapeutic frustrations; formulate unique insights; work through and "live through" the transference and countertransference and resistance and counterresistance; and develop other such therapeutic abilities. Ironically, this singular selfness is also the source for one's choice of neurosis and for one's neurotic choices.

The concept of a personal self—the "I"—in dynamic relation to an interpersonal self—the "me"—also profoundly affects the contemporary analyst's concept of the intersubjective, interpersonal field. For the more conservative coparticipant analyst, unique individuality remains implicit, and the therapeutic focus is on the interactive interplay between analyst and patient and their mutual impact on one another. In other words, field forces and dyadic adaptation—i.e., the interpersonal self—form the locus of therapeutic inquiry and study. In a sense, in this form of coparticipant inquiry the individual is reduced to the field. In a more comprehensive form of coparticipant inquiry involving the concept of a self-generative personal self, the individual strivings and understandings of the coparticipants are considered in a more complex way. Thus the individual is not reduced to the dyadic field and, unlike in Freudian clinical orthodoxy prior to the participant-observer model, the field is not reduced to the individual. In essence, coparticipant inquiry represents the clinical marriage of the interpersonal and personal selves—a synthesis of one-person and two-person psychologies; it is simultaneously cognizant of the individual and social dimensions of the psyches of both patient and analyst.

Thus, what defines coparticipant inquiry is not a specific clinical action or set of interventions, but rather a clinical attitude, an openness to the unique or singular, a profound sense of one's own and others' personal selfness. In coparticipant inquiry this sense of selfness, which we can know directly, immediate and unmediated, guides our analytic explorations and observations, which, in turn, result in consonant clinical actions, chosen spontaneously and specifically for the singular analytic moment.

The awareness of personal selfhood generally leads the analyst to look for patients' "openness to singularity" (see chapter 10) for evidence of originality and creativity or their inhibition. In parallel fashion, coparticipant analysts attend to their own openness (or closedness) to singularity. The concept of a personal self expands the clinical range of understanding and interpretation: there is a new openness to themes of the self's striving for personal fulfillment, both in narrative report and in analytic interaction. Previously, these efforts of the self would have gone unnoticed or mistakenly have been interpreted in terms of anxiety or loneliness (e.g., the self's striving for interpersonal approval and connection).

This brings us to the third principle of coparticipant inquiry—the concept of the patient as copartner.

THE PATIENT AS COPARTNER

In coparticipant inquiry patients are encouraged to fulfill their therapeutic interests, that is, to be analysts both of themselves and of their analysts. Therapeutic exploration, observation, confrontation, and interpretation are considered bidirectional and joint processes. For instance, if the coparticipant analyst were to ask the patient what he or she perceives about himself or herself or the analyst or some analytic event, this is not necessarily an effort to expand the transference—i.e., to have the patient articulate or enlarge upon his or her transference wishes or fears—as it would be in traditional psychoanalytic work or in the kind of transference analysis recommended by Merton Gill (1982a,b).

In coparticipant inquiry, the analyst may ask the patient what he or she thinks or feels primarily because the analyst values and wants to know the patient's singular understanding of the subject under discussion. In other words, the analyst's query is a genuine one, a true curiosity about the patient's unique perspective. At times this involves recognizing and encouraging the patients' desires, true and real, to analyze their analyst's countertransference in the immediate field of its occurrence. From a coparticipant perspective, analysts' questions of their patients' views of the countertransference are considered to be efforts to avail themselves of their patients' analytic abilities, rather than as an attempt to ferret out the transference plausibility of the patient's experience of his or her analytic coparticipation. Thus, the patient is seen as a therapeutic collaborator, capable of initiating or participating as a coequal in the mutual analysis of transference-countertransference impasses.

Acknowledging the patient as a copartner, in a true spirit of mutual analysis, tends to counter the problems of conceiving of the analyst as the omniscient "expert" doctor, which is a burden for both patient and analyst. In coparticipant inquiry the analyst is not required to single-handedly or omnipotently figure out everything or expertly execute a perfect technique. In contrast, coparticipant inquiry calls for a different concept of analytic expertise. Rather than assuming such traditional clinical roles as the interpretive surgeon or the all-knowing, mirroring parent or the expert participant interlocutor, the coparticipant analyst functions as an experiential guide, a coexplorer of the depths of the human psyche.

The analyst here is not *the* analytic "expert" with superior knowledge. Though the analyst should be knowledgeable and ideally also have gained some wisdom, he or she works more like a guide who facilitates the patient's development of his or her own metapsychological preferences and life directions. Helping the patient realize his own capacities for self-knowledge, the analyst participates in the growth of the patient's perspectives on life with others, which previously were anxiously avoided or simply unknown or unlived. Ideally, through their coparticipation, analysts serve as catalysts for the growth of the patient's autonomy—his or her sense of selfness. Patients, in turn, are free to make use of the analyst's expertise and wisdom as they wish and may incorporate aspects of the analyst's knowledge and understanding as they develop and follow their own truths.

Ideally, the coparticipant analyst helps to create analytic conditions—a safe and welcoming (and stimulating) psychological environment—within which patients can eventually let their defenses down, face their fears, and begin to recognize their curative and creative capacities. This process holds true for analysts as well—albeit in more subtle ways—as both regressive and progressive elements of their psychic life emerge in the therapy.

In sum, the notion of a personal self underlies true coparticipation. The coparticipant psychoanalytic perspective acknowledges patients' therapeutic capacities and their desire, no matter how well hidden, for analytic copartnership.

RESPONSIVITY AND RESPONSIBILITY

Therapeutic capability inevitably brings with it analytic responsibility. Patients are not only personally resourceful and, hopefully, interpersonally responsive (i.e., open to influence); they are also ultimately responsible for the success or failure of their therapy. The fourth defining feature of coparticipant analysis inheres in the coparticipant emphasis on patients' ultimate responsibility for their lives, their difficulties in living, for their analytic coparticipation and their personal growth—in short, for who they are and who they become.

In coparticipant inquiry analysts and patients are held accountable for their experience and desires, for generating their particular transferences or countertransferences, resistances and counterresistances (the analyst's resistances), and anxiety or counteranxiety (the analyst's anxiety). Each is also responsible for their shared inquiry into those experiences and desires and, ultimately, for working through and resolving them.

Coparticipant inquiry focuses on patients' personal responsibility for their therapy and their therapeutic experiences and actions, rather than limiting itself to the analytic effect or impact of the interpersonal other (i.e., the analyst). Coparticipant inquiry emphasizes patients' ability to heal themselves. No matter how hard they try or how well-intentioned or therapeutically talented they may be, analysts cannot *cure* patients; they can only *help* patients cure themselves. Sometimes they do this by not getting in the way of the patient and his or her unique way of help-ing or treating himself or herself.

Coparticipant inquiry is characterized by a corollary emphasis on patients' analytic strengths—their ability to reflect and to make mean-ingful psychological connections and constructions and on their striving toward mental health—their potential for mature relatedness. The copar-ticipant focus on patients' therapeutic capacities and on their attendant analytic responsibilities derives from the coparticipant emphasis on patients' sense of agency or personal selfness. Other psychoanalytic approaches also acknowledge the active and creative therapeutic role of the patient; however, they generally do not emphasize it to the degree that is characteristic of coparticipant inquiry. This takes us to another impor-tant characteristic of coparticipant inquiry, the fifth one in our list.

INDIVIDUATION OF METAPSYCHOLOGY AND METHODOLOGY

Given the uniqueness of patient and analyst and thus the uniqueness of their analytic relationship, it follows that coparticipant inquiry invites what Wolstein (1988) refers to as a radical individuation of psychoana-lytic metapsychologies (interpretive perspectives). As Wolstein observes,

> Every patient and every psychoanalyst is free . . . to pursue any inter-pretive and speculative outlook on metapsychology, old or new, that interests either or both of them. They may, for the first time, freely open the field and turn the procedure to the psychic uniqueness of their respective first-personal resources, arising from their unalien-able experience of the self in the active singular, private and public. . . . In fact . . . without both coparticipants, at some point, express-ing some uniquely individual slant on belief, value, and ideas, no psychoanalytic inquiry really takes hold. In sum, and this is the com-pelling direction in contemporary psychoanalytic inquiry, both coparticipants may suggest some uniquely individual emphasis in perspective on metapsychology, and select the particular myth and metaphor to depict their own private and closely held part in the clinical psychoanalytic inquiry. From this the following hypothesis emerges: that the number of uniquely individual perspectives now possible for interpretive usage in psychoanalytic metapsychology is practically infinite, no more, no less than the practically infinite number of coparticipants in the inquiry. (pp. 350–351)

An even more radical, and potentially liberating, implication of copartici-pation inheres in the complete individuation of methodologies; in other words, there is *no* right or proper or standard technique or form of analytic inquiry that fits all. This methodological pluralism, to my mind, represents one of the most radical features of the coparticipant approach to psychoanalytic practice. Historically, major theorists in clinical psychoanalysis have often formulated their preferred way of working analytically and then elevated this personal approach to an institutional level, claiming it was *the* correct way to work. Each analytic dyad, however, creates its own unique psychoanalytic situation and process. Each analyst and patient, in order to successfully complete their project, must figure out what they find to be personally and technically necessary to work with each other. From a coparticipant viewpoint there is no one standard or correct way to practice psychoanalysis that works for all psychoanalysts. Patients and analysts must create their own conditions for their joint inquiry into unconscious experience, their own and each other's.

However, finding one's own way does not mean that anything goes and that psychoanalytic discipline disappears and laziness and thoughtlessness rule the day. Rather, it means that there can be no rational canon of proper, prescribed techniques.

All analysts develop a body of generalizable clinical knowledge of psychopathology, clinical procedure, and analytic processes on the basis of their personal clinical experience in treating others or being treated themselves. And beyond their own experience, analysts also learn from their observation and study of the experiences of others. This cumulative clinical acumen or expertise informs analysts' understanding and treatment of all their patients—there is, in other words, methodological carryover from one situation to another. Generalizable and relevant, analysts' clinical knowledge is always applied to all of their work with all their patients, thus there is some measure of generality and similarity to their coparticipation in analysis. Nevertheless, each analytic dyad is unique, each analyst is unique, and each patient is unique—and so are the ways in which they work together. Wolstein (1987) summarizes this radical coparticipant perspective on psychoanalytic methodology (technique) when he points out that given the

> uniqueness of all psychoanalysts and patients, no one can claim supremacy in therapeutic inquiry for a preferred mode of procedure—which, in the final analysis, remains radically individual. . . .
> A psychoanalyst need not . . . adopt any one single attitude at all, and certainly not anyone else's, since the conduct of psychoanalytic inquiry is, in itself a matter of following one's deeply personal individual requirements. . . . The practical and viable recommendation to each psychoanalyst is: discover personal ways to best participate in clinical psychoanalytic inquiry. (pp. 336–337)

OPEN-ENDED CONCEPT OF INQUIRY

The coparticipant emphasis on unique ways of thinking and working calls for a bolder, freer, more "personal," and more spontaneous clinical approach than that generally characteristic of participant-observational approaches and of the impersonal technique advocated in the neoclassical textbooks. This open-ended concept of psychoanalytic inquiry forms the sixth defining clinical feature of the coparticipant approach.

Coparticipant inquiry comprises a continuum, from the conservative (more constrained or limited) to the more radical (more extreme or comprehensive) elaboration and application of this model of inquiry. Whether conservative or radical in their inquiry, coparticipant analysts vary in their individual ways of working. For example, some may use free association and a couch; others may pay more attention to the "here-and-now," use their countertransference experience, and may share more about themselves. Coparticipant analysts also differ in their attentiveness to regresssive material, in their uses of historical reconstruction, in their emphasis on extratransference issues, and so on. Nevertheless, those who practice from this paradigmatic perspective share a greater emphasis on self-expression and on self-disclosure—a more open sharing of experience—than can be found in more conventional forms of analytic inquiry.

Rejecting classical notions of analytic neutrality, anonymity, and abstinence, coparticipant analysts are characteristically active and expressive in their therapeutic use of themselves. They make active use of detailed inquiry, at times with directive and specific questioning in addition to—or in place of—traditional free-association. Coparticipant inquiry, as previously noted, is marked by a technical freedom for analytic self-disclosure and self-expression, including the judicious personal revelation and sharing of autobiographic facts, personal beliefs, and momentary emotional states. Accordingly, coparticipant analysts are more active and expressive in their therapeutic uses of countertransference experience than is typical of other analytic approaches.

Analysts who practice in a coparticipant way eschew the use of an analytic "persona"; such a concept goes against the very grain of coparticipant inquiry. Coparticipant analysts repudiate the classical notion of the analyst functioning like a blank screen or mirror and consider analytic anonymity a myth. Thus, they are not concerned with purifying the interpersonal field of analysis; from their coparticipant perspective, this is not only unnecessary but impossible. The analyst's personality is considered an integral part of the transference and inevitably revealed in it. Thus, the clinical focus of the coparticipant analyst is on the open examination of the countertransference by both analyst and patient, rather than on trying to constrain or legislate its inevitable emergence. Coparticipant analysts' active and expressive use of themselves does not imply a form of clinical impulsivity or "wild analysis." In contrast, coparticipant inquiry, given its radical field emphasis, mandates close attention to the transference and countertransference implications of analytic activity and an appreciation of the unique psychoanalytic perspectives of both coparticipants.

Coparticipant analysts recognize the clinical salience of analytic objectivity and nonintrusiveness. But respect for patients' motivational multidimensionality, psychic subjectivity, and need for analytic space cannot be guaranteed by prescription or mandated by analytic policy. Such an analytic attitude is guaranteed only by analysts' personal maturity and self-awareness and their openness to countertransference analysis. Only in this way is true analytic neutrality achieved—a neutrality of maturity, not one of analytic disengagement or of so-called objective monadic impersonality.

Coparticipant inquiry typically allows for a freer use of so-called analytic parameters than other analytic approaches. Though observant of the possible transference and countertransference ramifications of such interventions, coparticipant analysts are technically free to affirm, validate, educate, advise, sympathize with, reassure, comfort, confront, and otherwise intervene with their patients when such behavior is deemed therapeutically fruitful or clinically advisable. Coparticipant analysts are deeply mindful that the analytic process is, at heart, a human relationship, and they consider it an obligation to openly address and meet their patients' human needs for such so-called nonanalytic interventions. In general, coparticipant analysts regard the technical proscription of such active interventions as an institutionalized form of countertransference, one that forces analysts into covert and obscure expressions of such interventions, thus constraining or precluding their thoughtful observation.

Coparticipant inquiry calls for a more natural, less stilted and reserved way of interacting. It is less concerned with possibly impinging on the patient or with the strict observation of "the frame" of psychoanalytic exploration, particularly in its harshest, most rigid formulation, as it is exemplified in the reactionary yet strangely radical post-Freudian conceptions of Robert Langs (cf. 1975, 1982).

The coparticipant attitude emphasizes individual freedom and spontaneity and thus may be expressed and implemented in many different ways: some analysts are quiet, others garrulous; some are witty and openly playful, others more literal and serious; some are dramatic, others down-to-earth; some are slow and deliberate, others quick and intuitive, and so on. Analysts, like patients, come in many varieties; no two are identical. Though we are more alike than not—as Sullivan (1940) pointed out, we are also more unique than we think.

In contrast to the various forms of interpersonal participant-observation or impersonal nonparticipant-observation, coparticipant inquiry emphasizes the improvisatory nature of analytic work. Patient and analyst together develop new ways of working as new themes of inquiry or new clinical foci (such as, moving from a clinical focus on the extra-transference to a new emphasis on transference analysis) or urgent new clinical issues emerge in the inquiry. Coparticipant analysis focuses on analysis as a personal encounter, marked by experiences and events requiring an inquiry that arises organically from that unique relationship rather than from a book of analytic rules. The analytic process, when openly considered, proves to be an unpredictable process, with twists and turns, snags and starts, and motives and moves that neither of its coparticipant makers can predict. Thus, a spontaneous analytic treatment, if not proscribed or inhibited for personal or theoretical or political reasons, will largely prove to be an improvised experience. If inquiry is permitted to be open and is neither restricted nor controlled, but allowed to follow freely the emerging experience of its two coparticipants, it will develop in ways unexpected by both patient and analyst. Thus, coparticipant inquiry, in its emphasis on unique individuality, is marked by an improvisatory approach, rather than a literal following or methodical adapting of a prescribed canon of analytic technique.

However, the radical varieties of coparticipant inquiry are more improvisational than those that are more conservative. The many variations of coparticipant inquiry differ in important ways: one is the degree of freedom and openness allowed in clinical praxis. Radical coparticipation, which represents the consistent and comprehensive use of coparticipant principles, views the analytic relationship as a remarkably complex process whose therapeutic course and findings (results) are inherently unpredictable. In other words, we cannot know beforehand where an analytic investigation, will take the patient and his or her analyst. Improvisation and spontaneous responses are therefore indispensable. Those time-worn and tested technical rules shared and followed to some extent by all analysts may convey a sense of analytic order and method (which unquestionably has its place), but they can also, particularly when followed in an unthinking or slavish way, constrict the freshness, newness, and creative unpredictability of open-ended inquiry and improvisatory techniques. In its open-endedness and its rejection of a narrow technical canon and set of listening conventions, coparticipant inquiry expands the range of psychoanalytic practice and of therapeutic possibility.

Psychoanalytic inquiry is, or should be, what the term says: an inquiry, that is, a shared search, which by definition is born out of not (yet) know-ing the answers. This inquiry is thus always an experiment or exploration, a spontaneous trip into the heart of the unknown, a journey both unpre-dictable and uncertain. Faith in the human will to grow, to learn, and to know, gained from firsthand experience of one's selfness will mitigate the fear of such uncertainty and unpredictability. Such faith will also affirm the therapeutic potential of a radically open and free coparticipant inquiry and thus countermand the need for an authoritarian and impersonal methodology that is ultimately stultifying. The authoritarian approach develops generally as a defense against the anxiety and apprehension of encountering the unconscious and unknown depths of human passion, which emerges unpredictably in the coparticipant analytic process.

One may, in Fromm's phrase, seek to escape from freedom, to run from the frightening freedom of an open coparticipant inquiry and seek instead the comfort of a prescriptive and authoritarian technique. This search for order and authority, while perhaps pacifying some fears, inevitably forecloses the therapeutic promise of a deeply personal copar-ticipant inquiry: the possibility of true self-knowledge and its profoundly transformative potential. Coparticipant inquiry, when fully practiced, becomes an alive experience, deeply personal and fully connected; it is enlivening for both patient and analyst as they journey together into the heart of human feeling.

THE CURATIVE ROLE OF EXPERIENCE

The seventh feature defining coparticipant inquiry is its focus on the cur-ative role of immediate experience. Formulative hermeneutics is still regarded by coparticipant analysts as an integral and important part of psychoanalytic work, but it is not accorded the curative primacy it has in most psychoanalytic clinical theory and practice. This focus on the ana-lytic role of direct experience and the curative role of prelogical or pre-verbal experience is most pronounced in the practice of analysts follow-ing a comparatively radical form of coparticipant inquiry.

These analysts, usually affiliated with the interpersonal school, take to heart Sullivan's sardonic reminder that the supply of interpretations far exceeds the demand, and Thompson's simple reminder that what a patient needs is an *experience*, not an interpretation. These caveats refer, of course, to overly intellectualized approaches to analytic work and the excesses of interpretation, not the interpretive process per se. Yet, such cautions are in order, as a quick perusal of the analytic literature quickly reveals the highly intellectualized character of many analytic perspectives.

As presented in the contemporary literature, psychoanalytic treatment often seems heavily interpretive, overly concerned with the analyst's adverse influence on the patient (or, conversely, with the patient's adverse impact on the analyst), and preoccupied with an almost exquisite analysis of relational nuances, all this at the expense of a more down-to-earth experiential approach and humanistic view of human psychology. All too often the contemporary analytic literature seems abstruse and at times to lose sight of why patients seek treatment. Even among those who practice in a more coparticipant way there is a tendency to view patients (or patient-analyst interactions) as complicated assemblages of recondite psychodynamics, whether intrapsychic or interpsychic, as a set of complex dynamics to be analyzed in fine detail. What is missing is a view of the patient as a striving, suffering *person* interacting with another person in the hope (however hidden) of having a new and different and potentially liberating experience of himself or herself, an experience that is direct, singular, nonsymbolic, and concrete.

Coparticipant inquiry emphasizes the therapeutic role of immediate experience in two ways. First, there is a focus on the experiential dimension of the analyst-patient relationship and on the therapeutic potential of new experiences, new ways of thinking, feeling, and desiring that arise directly from the analytic relationship. This focus on the curative role of the analytic relationship, on what could be called reconstructive relational experience, has a long tradition in psychoanalytic history, originating in the coparticipatory concepts of Ferenczi. However, the therapeutic role of new relational experience has always, particularly among conservative traditional analysts, been rejected as nonanalytic. This problem stems from Alexander and French's (1946) original manipulative and mechanical conception of corrective emotional experience and the resulting fear among classical analysts that this would imply the centrality of suggestion in therapy and with that the potential for psychoanalysis to be dismissed as unscientific, its therapeutic effects the result of personal influence. The notion of a corrective emotional experience, however, won't go away. And that is because it contains a therapeutic truth—people get better when they are related to in new and healthier ways. (This is all discussed at greater length in the presentation of my concept of the "living through" process in chapter 13).

Benjamin Wolstein (1985, 1987, 1997) points to a second way in which direct experience—what may, in counterbalance to socially constructed syntaxic *interpretation*, be considered asocially constructed prototaxic or parataxic *experience*–plays an important therapeutic role.[2] According to Wolstein, it is in the individual's *direct, unmediated* experience of his or her emerging transference, resistance, anxiety, or psychic centeredness (i.e., sense of personal selfness) that awareness expands and change becomes possible. It is in this new, previously unconscious, experience, not in the application of personally preferred interpretive metaphor or myth, that one grows and changes. The patient has a new experience of himself or herself, instead of yet another interpretation, of which he or she has already had too many.

In a paper on the psychoanalysis of rage, Wolstein (1985) summarizes this coparticipant view of the therapeutic role of immediate experience as follows:

> Psychic knowledge of something unconscious becoming conscious we get only through the movement of immediate experience; and it gives us the kind of self-knowledge that no one can give to another. We come to understand such unique aspects of the self only during our own psychic movement of something unconscious into conscious awareness, from which arises that sense of self we name I. It is by going through this changing movement through immediate experience that we come to understand ourselves directly from within. Not for the self, but from it; in the active singular, first person. So we live and understand this sense of self in ways that subtend the inferential, conceptual, and highly symbolized formulations that others make of us, rationally coherent and logically correct though they may appear to be prior to our own self-knowledge gained through immediate experience. (pp. 624–625)

Further, Wolstein adds that patients

> all learn from others something about the adaptive-consensual meaning of rage, but only as they move into the experience themselves, undergo it and get through to its terminus, do they come to critically understand what it is for them first hand. . . . A patient works through rage, not as the psychoanalyst interprets it, but as the patient develops some unique understanding of the deeply held roots of this privately inflected experience. (pp. 622, 618)

It should be noted that immediate experience also plays a therapeutic role in generating intuitive processes of knowing, in unconscious or wordless communication with others, in creative self-expression, and in spontaneous action.

This, in brief, outlines the central features of coparticipant inquiry. These features are often present in varying degrees in the thought and work of analysts who generally follow other analytic approaches. Moreover, analysts may selectively—though not necessarily consciously—practice according to coparticipant principles in some situations and not others. For example, they may follow those principles with some patients but not others, with some analytic issues or themes but not others, and so on. Nevertheless, to the degree that an analyst (or patient) lives out the qualities of inquiry outlined here, to that degree that analyst (or patient) can be justifiably considered to pursue a coparticipant inquiry.

Coparticipant inquiry is probably best defined, and best known to its practitioners, in the direct experience of its clinical application, that is, by doing it. Coparticipant inquiry carries the live potential for a free, creative, and open relatedness to one's analytic copartner and to oneself. It is, or can be, an enlivening, even exhilarating experience. Of course, this potential may be repudiated, defended against, dissociated, or selectively ignored because of emerging apprehension, anxiety or shame about being fully alive. The analyst, out of his or her unconscious needs and fears, may need to find some other, more comfortable, less frightening way to work, perhaps retaining those aspects of coparticipant practice that are not perceived as frightening.

Analysts, like most people, often fear experiences of uniqueness and mutuality. Many analysts, anxious about thinking out and upholding their own original ideas of metapsychology and methodology, seek relief by borrowing, at times slavishly, some prominent analyst's ideas and ways of working. Fearful of working in their unique way, or coordinating their way with the patient's unique way, these analysts often search and long for an omnipotent authority, for some universally applicable technique and metapsychology, so as not to have to reach for their own original way of working with others and understanding them.

Analysts and patients also may fear not only their own uniqueness but also the mutuality and intimacy that arise in a coparticipant way of working. Some prefer to repudiate and avoid getting really close, both to their own self and to the other. And therefore many retreat, temporarily or permanently, to a less personal coparticipatory technique.

It is interesting to note that mutuality arises necessarily when the individuals involved are most fully individuated since only then are they capable of an open, mature give-and-take. This is a mutuality of peers, kindred souls, not a defensive mutual adaptation to each other's insecurities. It is a true meeting, neither insecure nor defensive, of two people coming together, each acting, feeling, and thinking in self-realized terms. Such moments in analysis, as in life, are transforming.

Let us now consider, at greater length, the history of coparticipant inquiry in the evolution of psychoanalytic praxis.

CHAPTER 3

The Evolution of Coparticipant
Inquiry in Psychoanalysis

It begins with Freud; in his work we find the first hints of a coparticipant analytic sensibility. By nature an explorer, bold and incisive, passionately committed to the search for psychological truth, to exploring the depths of the human soul, Freud evidenced an early sense of the coparticipatory nature of the clinical analytic encounter. However, encumbered by a nagging fear that his creation, psychoanalysis, would be dismissed as unscientific, its therapeutic benefit solely the result of suggestion rather than the objective result of scientific procedure and methodology, Freud highlighted the aspect of objective *nonparticipant observation* of his method. In response to the mechanistic objectivity and positivism of his intellectual milieu and impressed with the adaptational Darwinism of his day, Freud chose to de-emphasize the spontaneity and reciprocity of the coparticipant encounter. After focusing instead on the role of the psychoanalyst as that of an "objective" *nonparticipant observer*, the analyst thus became the expert whose surgical interpretations laid bare patients' neurotic secret lives and the workings of their unconscious inner worlds.

According to firsthand reports, Freud himself worked in a highly active manner, and patients often experienced him as authoritarian and opinionated. He has been described as a "vivid and even argumentative therapist" (Bergmann 1976, p. 28). In at least one instance he fed and even lent money to a patient. Freud was a pragmatic clinician and his therapeutic efforts at times crossed what today's orthodox analysts would consider proper analytic boundaries. This highly interactive and personal method of treatment stands in sharp contrast to Freud's conservative and cautious prescription for a sturdy and emotionally austere psychoanalysis based on the principles of analytic abstinence, clinical neutrality, and therapeutic anonymity (the analyst as blank screen).

In his recommendations on analytic technique, Freud (1910a,b; 1912a,b; 1913; 1914a; 1915; 1937) called for an objective and impersonal, or *nonparticipant*, methodology. Freud's recommendations on psychoanalytic technique, tailored to fit his personality and cultural milieu, were taken to the extreme and turned illogical and countertherapeutic in the purist practices of orthodox American Freudian analysts of the mid-twentieth century. This austere and often harsh misreading of classical technique showed little of Freud's own exploratory spirit and human(e) therapeutic activity.

Though taken to an absurd and countertherapeutic level by those who lacked Freud's spirited sense of analytic encounter, many of his technical recommendations dating from the early 1900s have proven to be of lasting value. For example, the classical focus on analysts being as objective or impartial as possible in their clinical judgments has had lasting therapeutic importance. Similarly, the analytic merit of nonintrusiveness and noninterference with analysts' or patients' ongoing creative or autonomous psychic processes is implicit in the principle of evenly listening to the patient's free association. Moreover, the principle of analytic neutrality addresses the clinical ideal of being nonjudgmental. The principle of neutrality points also to the therapeutic significance of allowing patients to mirror themselves in analytic monologue. These classical technical concepts still constitute useful and important aspects of contemporary psychoanalytic therapy. For Freud they represented important indices and reflections of a scientific methodology, which was of vital importance to his view of the "future prospects of psycho-analytic therapy" (Freud 1910a)

However, these early principles of psychoanalytic conduct also have a darker potential: they can be construed in overly narrow, literal, and dogmatic ways, as conservative and orthodox Freudian analysts did from the early 1920s to today. Such authoritarian and impersonal practice, however, was most characteristic of the analytic practices of American Freudian analysts from the 1920s through the 1950s. Many of these analysts worked within a highly circumscribed set of rigid, authoritarian rules that led to a harsh quasi-rigorous and pseudoscientific methodology that was often countertherapeutic in its impact. Leo Stone (1961), among other moderate Freudians, offered a detailed and reasoned critique of such misguided impersonal concepts of the psychoanalytic situation. A traditional and more moderate version of Freudian psychoanalysis is articulated by Greenson (1967). (See also Brenner [1976] and Menninger [1958] for contemporary texts on conservative, *nonparticipant* forms of

Freudian psychoanalysis. More modern *coparticipant* forms of Freudian psychoanalysis are considered later in this chapter.)

In the markedly conservative approach of the orthodox Freudians of the 1920s to the 1950s psychoanalysis was marked by the noninteractive stance, emotional constriction, affective remoteness, and long analytic silences of the *nonparticipant* analyst. This analytic situation often approached the caricature of the enigmatic, laconic analyst locked in silent psychic battle with his or her mute and resistant patient. In actuality such silences were often punctuated by terse (or sometimes lengthy) interpretations. All too often, they represented unimaginative applications of presumed universal truths, formulaic metapsychological pronouncements, or authoritarian ex cathedra fiats. In this analytic perspective the patient becomes the passive recipient of the analyst's interpretive "surgery": the detached, neutral analyst opens the *nonparticipant* patient to his or her libidinal truths.

In contrast to such narrow orthodox analytic perspectives and readings of Freud, modern coparticipant analytic perspectives find new and broader meanings in Freud's principles of analytic inquiry. For instance, the traditional analytic principle of anonymity (the blank screen or mirror) was once thought indispensable therapeutically, but analytic anonymity is now largely seen as therapeutically unnecessary, and as impossible to achieve. In fact, one can understand the theory of analytic anonymity as an institutionalized form of counterresistance, a defensive refusal to acknowledge the interaction that flows continuously between patient and analyst. Thus the principle of analytic anonymity, ostensibly developed or adopted to provide analytic space for the transference to freely show itself unimpeded by the analyst's personal issues, may actually be used defensively to justify analysts' fearful avoidance of their potentially intimate connection with their patients.

For many analysts, Freud's therapeutic recommendations define standard or classical psychoanalytic technique; even when taken to extremes, these principles still represent the true standard for psychoanalytic inquiry and analytic conduct. These conservative analytic approaches still define the impersonal *nonparticipant* paradigm of psychological inquiry even today.

There is no coparticipant inquiry to be found in these analytic approaches; here, patients are not considered active and proactive collaborators or copartners, able to choose, to will, and to inquire about themselves and also about their analysts. Post-Freudians, with their austere and authoritarian exaggeration of Freud's technical precepts and recommendations, have shown little interest in coparticipant approaches.

Yet, one can see sparks of a coparticipant sensibility in the clinical approach and work of Freud and some of his early disciples. According to many reports, including firsthand reports by former patients, Freud clearly was an active, lively, interactive (and authoritarian) analytic participant, and if he were alive today, he might well practice in a manner I call coparticipant. In any event, Freud practiced in a way that differed considerably from the procedure he advised. In Freud's writings one finds the occasional brief glimpse of a coparticipant sensibility, the faint beginnings of what would eventually develop into coparticipant inquiry.

The following remarks Freud wrote in 1912 in the first of his series of papers on psychoanalytic therapy are an illustrative example:

> The technical rules which I bring forward here have been evolved out of my own experience in the course of many years, after I had renounced other methods which had cost me dear. . . . My hope is that compliance with them will spare physicians practicing analysis much unavailing effort. . . . I must, however, expressly state that this technique has proved to be the only method suited to my individuality; I do not venture to deny that a physician quite differently constituted might feel impelled to adopt a different attitude to his patients and to the task before him. (1912a, p. 323)

Freud here points explicitly to the interpersonal uniqueness of every analytic situation and the personal uniqueness of every analyst, including himself. This is a cornerstone of coparticipant inquiry. Freud, however, was far from holding or recommending a coparticipatory view of the psychoanalytic situation (see p. 45 for a schematic adjectival comparison of the *nonparticipant* and the *coparticipant* paradigms). In Freud's traditional and authoritarian view, analysts are neither infallible nor omniscient (nor omnipotent); however, they are still thought to know better than the suffering patient what his or her problems are and what is therapeutically best for him or her.

Nevertheless, there are signs here of a coparticipatory analytic sensibility, as can be seen in the following comments from Freud's early (1910a) paper on the "future prospects of psychoanalytic therapy":

> We have begun to consider the "counter-transference," that arises in the physician as a result of the patient's influence on his unconscious feelings, and have nearly come to the point of requiring the physician to recognize and overcome this counter-transference in himself. (p. 289)

Freud tells us further that the analyst

> must bend his own unconscious like a receptive organ towards the emerging unconscious of the patient, be as the receiver of the telephone

to the disc. As the receiver transmutes the electric vibrations induced by the sound-waves back again into sound-waves, so is the physician's unconscious mind able to reconstruct the patient's unconscious, which has directed his associations, from the communications derived from it. (1912b, p. 328)

We see here an allusion to mutual analytic influence and to unconscious dialogue, themes Ferenczi was to develop later. Freud implicitly touches here, perhaps inadvertently, on another cornerstone of coparticipant inquiry, the fundamentally interpersonal character or field nature of the analytic situation.

Despite these early traces of a coparticipant sensibility, Freud, for the reasons noted earlier, shrunk from pursuing coparticipant inquiry and its bidirectional implications. He retreated from any notion of analytic mutuality to an authoritarian, one-way concept of analytic inquiry. Although countertransference is implicitly seen as an interpersonal phenomenon, Freud remained steadfast in his hierarchical and monadic approach to the analysis of transference and countertransference. There is no hint here of a possible coparticipant analysis of the analyst's subjective experience. Despite tendencies to the contrary, Freud eschewed an interpersonal view of the analytic situation. He did not develop the coparticipatory implications of his own highly interactive clinical work. Instead, Freud viewed the analyst as a nonparticipant mirror or, to use another of his metaphors, an impersonal psychic surgeon. As Freud (1912b) put it,

I cannot recommend my colleagues emphatically enough to take as a model in psycho-analytic treatment the surgeon who puts aside all his own feelings, including that of human sympathy, and concentrates his mind on one single purpose, that of performing the operation as skillfully as possible. . . . The physician should be impenetrable to the patient, and, like a mirror, reflect nothing but what is shown to him. (pp. 327, 331)

Freud writes here of the quintessential nonparticipant expert analyst. We see in Freud's own practice and in his recommendations and guidelines for praxis the signs of participatory theory—the dim outlines of a more participatory perspective on the psychoanalytic process. Nevertheless, Freud never defined the analyst as a *participant-observer* or as a *coparticipant inquirer*. Freud's analyst, at least in theory if not in practice, remains the impersonal and expert psycho-surgeon, the reflecting mirror, objective and *nonparticipant* interpreter of the other. (See table 3.1.)

Table 3.1 Comparison of Nonparticipant and Coparticipant Paradigms

Nonparticipant (Classical or Standard Technique)	Coparticipant
prescriptive	Improvisatory
Authoritarian	Egalitarian
One-way	Two-way
Intrapsychic	Intra- and interpsychic
One-person psychology	One-person and two-person psychology
Encapsulated psyche	Interactive or intersubjective field
Rigid	Flexible
Restrictive (nonintrusive)	Freer technique (engaging)
Controlling	Confrontative
Monistic (one right way)	Pluralistic (many right ways)
Universals	Uniqueness
Free-associative	Free and focused attention
Hermeneutic focus (on interpretation)	Relational focus (on immediate experience)
Verbal emphasis	Actional emphasis
Anonymity (limited self-disclosure)	Openness to self-disclosure
Prescribed neutrality	Chosen impartiality
Blank screen	Open revelation
Hierarchical	Collaborative mutuality
Traditional	Experimental
Defined and circumscribed role of analyst	Analyst free to develop own methodology
Generally silent analyst	Analyst silent and/or talking
Interpretive insight curative	Curative "living through"
Nonintrusiveness	Risks engagement

FERENCZI: THE FIRST COPARTICIPANT ANALYST

It was Sandor Ferenczi, the spirited Hungarian analyst and *enfant terrible* of psychoanalysis, who in his clinical experiments with new forms of psychoanalytic inquiry first openly practiced what essentially was a radical (i.e., extreme) form of coparticipant inquiry. Considered by many to have been the most brilliant and intuitive of Freud's inner circle, Ferenczi's courageous questioning of the orthodox precepts of classical psychoanalytic praxis and his creative efforts to develop a more experiential and mutually exploratory inquiry mark the beginnings of coparticipant psychoanalysis.

Though a devoted disciple, friend, and former analysand of Freud, Ferenczi, rebellious and revolutionary in spirit, was motivated to experiment with more active modes of psychoanalytic inquiry and intervention. Ferenczi experimented with a radically new, active, and at times, directive analytic inquiry. This had three forms, which he called the active method, the relaxation technique, and the most radical of all, mutual analysis.

Ferenczi's experiments in modified psychoanalysis (Ferenczi 1916, 1926) began with his ill-fated attempt to carry out Freud's analytic rule of abstinence. Ferenczi hypothesized that strictly prohibiting patients' libidinal gratification, not only in analysis but also in their everyday lives, would augment psychic tensions and thus facilitate the therapeutic work. This psychoanalytic version of "tough love," of prescribed deprivation, aroused considerable feelings of irritation and rage, as might be expected. This iatrogenically born negativity, a natural reaction to such psychic constriction, doomed Ferenczi's ill-considered experiment. As for coparticipant inquiry, there was nothing coparticipant in any of this.

Yet, in Ferenczi's search for a better and more therapeutic analytic approach—in his very willingness to go beyond analytic orthodoxy in order to find a more effective and active therapy—we see the seeds of a coparticipant sensibility that was to flower in his radically innovative concept of mutual analysis and his novel technique of analytic relaxation or indulgence.

Though clearly ahead of their time, Ferenczi's radical experiments with coparticipant concepts of analytic inquiry were, as he himself acknowledged, flawed and ultimately unworkable. Nevertheless, they represent a bold, imaginative leap from a passive and authoritarian therapy to an egalitarian, two-way form of inquiry that prefigured what would eventually evolve into a coparticipant psychoanalysis. In contrast to the intellectualized formality, artificial neutrality, and technical rigidity of the analytic orthodoxy of his day, Ferenczi's bold experiments showed the way to a freer, more human, and more interactive, field-oriented coparticipant analytic inquiry. As Stanton (1991) points out, Ferenczi was sharply critical of orthodox

> psychoanalyst inactivity which justified itself by appeal to scientific objectivity and neutrality. In his view, severely regressed patients did not need guarantees of the scientific integrity of the analyst's interpretations, but genuine affective support and nourishment. In some cases, this meant active intervention, such as recommendations and prohibitions. . . . In others, it meant soothing, relaxing and even touching the patient. (p. 76)

Ferenczi's empiricism and his effort to develop a true coparticipant base for analytic technique have borne fruit in the coparticipant ideas and work of succeeding generations of analysts, particularly those who have identified themselves with contemporary interpersonal, object relations, and intersubjective conceptions of analytic therapy.

In his formulation of the relaxation technique and principle of indulgence, Ferenczi argued for a friendlier and more open and flexible analytic situation. Critical of orthodoxy's intellectualized interpretive approach and its austere analytic procedures, rules, and conditions, which he thought contributed to the sterility of many analytic relationships and to a diminishing sense of psychoanalytic effectiveness, Ferenczi believed that psychoanalysis was nearing a dead end therapeutically (cf. Thompson 1958). This was, in part, the motivating force behind Ferenczi and Rank's (1925) search for a more effective and experientially oriented form of analysis, and it led to their monograph on developments in psychoanalytic praxis. Rank, like Ferenczi, demonstrated a coparticipant sensibility. However, unlike Ferenczi, he broke with Freud's metapsychology. Advocating his own theory of personality and psychopathology, Rank went his own independent way, much to Freud's distress (cf. Monroe 1955; Menaker 1982).

Ferenczi's notion of neocatharsis and the relaxation technique reflected his belief that instead of ever more interpretations (and their potential for theoretical indoctrination) patients need a new experience, particularly new experiences of "love." Rather than striving for intellectual understanding, analysts, according to Ferenczi, need to provide analytic tenderness, on both the psychological and the physical level. Ferenczi believed that patients suffer from a lack of love (perhaps a projection of his own deep want) in the nonerotic, parental sense, and the analyst must provide it so that a therapeutic change could take place.

The boldness and experimental quality of his work as well as Ferenczi's willingness to create innovative and individualized approaches, rather than the specific method of conveying love, marks this approach as coparticipant in spirit. Though I believe that Ferenczi was essentially correct in his assessment of patients' needs for love—for tenderness, care, concern, respect, empathy, sympathy, and the like—there is some question about the therapeutic implications of consistent, prescribed physical touch. Of course, Freud was dismayed by Ferenczi's therapeutic experiments. In a famous letter he took Ferenczi to task for his new "kissing technique." Ferenczi defended his new, more liberal view of the analytic situation and in turn criticized Freud's approach. Whatever merits or therapeutic implications the relaxation technique offered, it framed a central psychoanalytic controversy that continues unabated to this day, namely, the question of whether and to what degree people change because of interpretive insight or new interpersonal experiences.

As was to be expected, Freud found the third form of active analytic intervention, mutual analysis, even harder to accept than Ferenczi's deprivation method or indulgence technique. Though flawed and ultimately unworkable as practiced, Ferenczi's ([1931]1988) experiments with mutual analysis (in which analyst and patient alternated as therapist) definitely moved his thinking and practice in a radically coparticipant direction.

Haynal (1996) observes that

> Diverging increasingly from Freud, Ferenczi came close to a new conception, a sort of field theory that anticipates later developments in psychoanalysis, at a time when the basis of field theory . . . had not yet been laid. (p. 36)

Stanton (1991) similarly notes that Ferenczi's analytic

> paradigm is an anarchic "mutual aid": it replaces the one-way process in which the analyst observes, then offers a diagnosis of the patient, with a two-way co-operative dialogue.
>
> Without appreciating, or judging, either "active" or "mutual" analysis, . . . it is important to see how they shift the analytical balance from transference to countertransference. Ferenczi insists that the two cannot be separated. The analyst's interpretations cannot be immunized from countertransferential elements, which in turn need to be analyzed at some point for patients, that is, in relation to their transference. The supervision of analytical sessions is therefore essential, but does not remove the responsibility of bringing the countertransference into the analytical process itself. (p. 62)

Ferenczi's trial of mutual analysis with his now famous patient, R. N. (which actually was a form of alternating analyses) was marked by an analytic openness to mutual influence and individuality of experience, a clinical emphasis on immediate experience, a spirit of egalitarianism and a repudiation of traditional analytic authority, and by clinical boldness and freedom of inquiry. Ferenczi's innovativeness, experimental sensibility, concepts of analytic mutuality, honesty, equality, and openness, and his respect for unique individuality identify his work and clinical approach as strongly coparticipant. His concept of mutual analysis actually represents a far more radical form of coparticipant inquiry than that practiced by most contemporary analysts (Ferenczi 1916, 1926, 1931).

Ferenczi's teachings, particularly as they have been advanced by such influential analysands and students as Michael Balint, Melanie Klein, Franz Alexander, and Clara Thompson, have had a profound impact on the British schools of object-relations and the American school of interpersonal relations, both of which in recent years have developed coparticipant notions of psychoanalytic praxis. Ferenczi's clinical ideas were an important contribution to that vast and momentous shift in psychoanalytic thought and practice that I call the *interpersonal turn*.

This interpersonal or relational turn describes the evolutionary shift from an impersonal therapy and biological drive theory (metapsychology) to an interpersonal (and eventually personal) therapy and social personality theory. Ferenczi's contribution to this sea change in psychoanalytic perspective was a major one. His exploratory spirit, interpersonal sensibility, and courageous clinical experiments were vitally important to the development of the second clinical psychoanalytic paradigm—*participant-observation,* out of which the third paradigm, *coparticipant inquiry,* has gradually emerged.

In one respect Ferenczi, unlike some first-generation analysts of Freud's inner circle, never left Freud—he never questioned the libido theory, Freud's metapsychological creation. Unlike the early dissidents Adler, Jung, and Rank, Ferenczi never challenged the universality or primacy of Freud's preferred view of the human psyche. Ferenczi was first and foremost a therapist, a healer, and interested primarily in the specifics of helping others. Freud, by contrast, was first and foremost a psychological explorer or investigator, a researcher, and interested primarily in understanding the universals of the human mind.

Ferenczi's major contribution to psychoanalysis was his radical and far-reaching proposal for restructuring the nature of the psychoanalytic situation and method along the lines he recommended, anticipating in this many of the interpersonal and object-relations approaches to clinical work that followed. Many of our contemporary psychoanalytic controversies about questions of analytic authority, autonomy, and authenticity, about the nature of therapeutic action in psychoanalysis, about the dilemmas of self-disclosure and expressive uses of countertransference, and about the optimal definition of analytic boundaries are foreshadowed in the controversial clinical findings of Sandor Ferenczi, the first coparticipant analyst.

Ferenczi's search for a mutual analysis was motivated by deep personal as well as professional reasons. As Fortune (1996) points out, "mutual analysis was, in part, Ferenczi's response to his own unresolved transference-countertransference issues with Freud" (p. 178). It formed "a part of Ferenczi's . . . struggle to clarify his enmeshed and ambivalent relationship to Freud" (p.179). Ferenczi blamed his analyst for failing to analyze his negative transference and for failing to love him. Judith Dupont, Ferenczian scholar and editor of his *Clinical Diary* ([1931]/1988), astutely observes that as both analyst and analysand, Ferenczi, experienced firsthand

> The shortcomings of the so-called classic techniques. . . . In the criticisms directed at him by his patients, he recognizes his own criticisms formulated to Freud. He endeavors to invent for his patients

what he wanted Freud to invent for him. He tries to offer them the understanding and trust that he himself had been unable to obtain from Freud. . . . When he reproaches Freud for having construed the analytic situation so as to assure above all the protection and comfort of the analyst, he is in fact reproaching him for refusing to listen when what he, Ferenczi, is saying threatens Freud's own internal security. . . . Ferenczi dares to hear and dares to express feelings, ideas, intuitions, and sensations that generally have great difficulty working their way to consciousness and even greater difficulty allowing themselves to be formulated in words. . . . He thus opens to psychoanalysts . . . new directions . . . bringing a healthy and invigorating breath of fresh air in those places . . . where the theories and technical principles of psychoanalysts have a tendency to settle and to become fixed. (Ferenczi/Dupont, [1931]/1988, p. xxvi)

INTERPERSONAL PSYCHOANALYSIS AND COPARTICIPANT INQUIRY

Concepts of participant-observation and coparticipant inquiry began to take hold in the work of many psychoanalytic clinicians in the 1920s and 1930s, except for the staunchly orthodox analysts. This *interpersonal turn* in psychoanalysis represented an almost tectonic shift from a drive metapsychology and an impersonal technique to a relational metapsychology and an interpersonal theory of inquiry.

The rising theoretical influence of the American school of interpersonal relations and the British school(s) of object-relations tilted psychoanalytic study toward relational and interpersonal concepts of praxis and away from classical thought and practice. Particularly crucial was Harry Stack Sullivan's groundbreaking formulation of the psychoanalytic situation as an *interpersonal field* in which the analyst is inevitably a *participant-observer*. Although interpersonal psychoanalysis has made an important contribution to the development of psychoanalytic theory, it has had a deeper impact on psychoanalytic practice.

Historically, the American school has shared with British object-relations theory and post-Freudian ego-psychology a common clinical focus on character (ego) analysis, the analysis of the self in all its multidimensionality, and the use of techniques modified for the analysis of the severely disturbed. Though these cognate schools of thought and practice share a view of the analytic situation as an interpersonal (intersubjective) process, the American school has been a more radical one; unlike the British school, post-Freudian ego analysis, and the more recent self-psychology, it bears no ties, in either spirit or language, to orthodox psychoanalytic theory.

Like its coevals—the post-Freudian ego-analytic and British schools—the American school has developed into a rich, complex, and diverse school, encompassing a wide variety of theoretical viewpoints and clinical practices. The American interpersonal school, given its pragmatic outlook, perspectivism, and clinical open-endedness, is home to a greater diversity of clinical thought and practice than any other psychoanalytic school. The interpersonal approach has had a pervasive, though largely unacknowledged, influence on psychoanalytic praxis and theory; many interpersonal concepts and practices have been silently adopted by mainstream psychoanalysis.

Among the numerous features of the interpersonal approach that have been instrumental in facilitating the evolution of the coparticipant perspective in psychoanalytic praxis are its characteristic pragmatic emphasis on workability, its egalitarian spirit, its flexibility in technique and field-theory orientation, and its interactive and empirical emphasis on actual experience in psychic functioning. The most important feature of interpersonal psychoanalysis for evolving concepts of coparticipant inquiry is its conception of the analytic situation as an interpersonal field, originally framed in terms of Sullivan's principle of participant-observation.

The principle of participant-observation, as articulated by Sullivan, was pivotal in the evolution of clinical psychoanalysis. Patient and analyst would from now on be seen as participating in a mutual experiential field. The analyst, no longer a nonparticipant mirror, was now a participant-observer, an active factor in what he or she would observe. This seminal concept is tied to Sullivan's other major therapeutic concepts, such as the disjunctive role of anxiety, the resistance of the self-system's security (i.e., defensive) operations, and the clinical primacy of the analysis of the interpersonal self. Sullivan's participant-observer differed greatly from Freud's mirror-analyst and signaled a significant shift in psychoanalytic technique, which now included a detailed, focused inquiry in addition to free association, a method many interpersonalists regard as therapeutically inefficient.

According to Sullivan, psychopathology originates in the experience of anxiety, the sudden, terrifying drop in self-esteem occasioned by social disapproval. As is discussed further in chapter 4, Sullivan considered anxiety to be interpersonal, originally "caught" or induced through empathic processes from significant others. In Sullivan's theoretical schema, the inner interpersonal world of mental representations, or "personifications" of oneself and others (the myriad states of good-me, bad-me, and not-me), is the psychic derivative of the human need to distinguish anxious from nonanxious experience. Thus, for Sullivan, the self was the sum of reflected appraisals—the sum of approvals from significant others. It was this interpersonal dimension of the self and its vicissitudes that most captured Sullivan's clinical attention.

Like modern intersubjectivists, Sullivan thought that people could be understood only contextually; that is, what patients say makes sense only when understood in participatory terms. Sullivan even went so far as to define personality in dyadic (or polyadic) terms as the "relatively enduring pattern of recurrent interpersonal situations which characterize a human life" (1953, p. 111). In other words, humans are inherently communal; we all are born into a society of others, each of us destined to live life bounded by our attachments.

When the analyst is a participant-observer rather than the classically defined nonparticipant mirror, this has clear implications for the interpersonal view of the psychoanalytic process, including the analysis of transferential phenomena. First of all, it recognizes the perspectival nature of the analytic situation; the analytic observer, whether patient or analyst, inevitably will see the other (and himself or herself) from some personal perspective. In other words, an observational stance of neutrality is not possible (Wolstein 1959, 1977; Levenson 1972, 1983; Singer 1965; Ehrenberg 1992; Hoffman 1983; Stern 1997). Perhaps even more important, however, is the interactional principle inherent in the concept of participant-observation: in the act of observing, the observer inevitably affects the observed, and the observed inevitably affects the participant-observer's observing. In other words, transference and countertransference are jointly generated: they are inevitably field processes, reciprocal aspects of an interactive, experiential field. The analyst is not, and cannot be, a blank screen (Thompson 1950; Will 1954; Wolstein 1954, 1977a,b; Singer 1965; Searles 1965; Crowley 1952, 1977; Cohen 1953; Hoffman 1983; Hirsch 1987; Fiscalini 1995a,b; Stern 1992, 1997).

From this conception of the analytic situation as an interpersonal field derives the interpersonal view of transference and countertransferences as compresent and interpenetrating field processes (Wolstein 1959; Levenson 1972; Tauber 1954, 1979; Epstein and Feiner 1979; Fiscalini 1995a,b; Hirsch 1996. From a contemporary coparticipant perspective, every analytic dyad is seen as generating its own interpersonal and unique transference-countertransference matrix of action and experience (Wolstein 1988; Marshall and Marshall 1988; Bass 2001a). An important clinical implication of this field concept of transference and countertransference is that understanding the patient's personality inevitably involves an understanding of the analyst's personality.

From this participant-observer perspective, analytic expertise inheres in the ability to observe and appraise one's inevitable participation with patients. As Sullivan (1949) sardonically put it, psychoanalytic expertise refers to the analyst's "skill in participant observation in the unfortunate patterns of his own and the patient's living, in contrast to merely participating in such unfortunate patterns with the patient" (p. 12).

Sullivan's formulations imply the clinical reciprocity of transference and countertransference patterns and the clinical centrality of their coordinated inquiry. This coparticipant possibility has been elaborated and developed by such interpersonal theorists as Edgar Levenson, Warren Wilner, and Benjamin Wolstein as well as by some relationists, such as Lewis Aron, Anthony Bass, and the late Stephen Mitchell.

From Sullivan's view of the analyst as an expert participant-observer it follows that the inquiring analyst "has an inescapable, inextricable involvement in all that goes on in the [analytic] interview" and that analysts "should never lose track of the fact that all the processes of the patient are more or less exactly addressed" (1954, p. 19) to them and vice-versa.

Over the years, many interpersonalists have extended Sullivan's participant-observer concept in directions not anticipated by Sullivan (see, for example, Thompson 1956; Tauber 1954; Wolstein 1954, 1959, 1988; Levenson 1972, 1982b, 1985; Epstein and Feiner 1979; and Feiner 1979, 1988, 1991). Building upon Sullivan's seminal interpersonal insights, these interpersonal analysts began to revise Sullivan's participant conception of analytic observation with more extensive and comprehensive concepts of a coparticipatory praxis. Possessing a keen understanding of the coparticipant nature of analytic experience, such seminal interpersonal analysts as Levenson (1972), Tauber and Green (1959, 1979), and Wolstein (1954, 1959, 1977a, 1983a,b, 1997) began as early as the 1950s to recommend what then were radical steps toward a reformation of psychoanalytic practice in the direction of a more open and comprehensive coparticipant inquiry. These theorists advocated, for example, coparticipant practices such as the explicit sharing of analysts' prelogical associational experience or countertransference experience, including the open sharing of analysts' dreams of their patients (Tauber). They also supported treating transference and countertransference as naturally co-created and indivisible continua of irrational or nonrational experience (Wolstein) and the open encouragement of the mutual analysis of countertransference in the analytic field of its origin (Wolstein). They argued that analysts, even in their interpretive duties, are inevitably "transformed" by their patients, for example, subtly provoked to reenact old patterns of relatedness, so-called transference-countertransference enactments (Levenson). These expanded conceptions of the interpersonal field were significantly influenced not only by Sullivan's interpersonal concepts but also by the experientialist and humanistically oriented interpersonal work of Fromm.

Fromm thought that Sullivan had not gone far enough in redefining the analyst's participatory role and suggested that the analyst's role was that of an "observant participant" rather than that of a "participant observer."[1] Fromm advanced his understanding of the analytic relationship as a personal human encounter—ideally one marked by a spontaneous experience of authentic "core-to-core" relatedness between patient and analyst. Fromm thus called for a confrontative therapy aimed at cutting through cerebration to an immediate experience of psychic reality.

Fromm's view of the psychoanalytic situation as one of participatory engagement and open encounter has influenced subsequent interpersonalists' clinical work, and it forms one of the major roots of current interpersonal concepts of coparticipant inquiry. Fromm's focus on the active participatory nature of the analytic relationship has been elaborated by more recent generations of interpersonal analysts (such as Arthur Feiner, Edgar Levenson, Edward Tauber, and Benjamin Wolstein) into contemporary formulations of clinical psychoanalysis in radical coparticipant terms.

Sullivan's theory of the analyst as participant-observer presents a striking irony. Sullivan brought to psychoanalysis the concept of an interpersonal analytic field, but he did not work in the transference or the countertransference, at least not in any comprehensive or consistent way. Ironically, it was Freud, the advocate of a nonparticipant concept of analytic inquiry, who emphasized the importance of working in the transference.[2]

In his emphasis on extratransference inquiry, on working outside of the "here and now" transference-countertransference field, Sullivan failed to develop the radical implications of his own seminal conception of the interpersonal analytic field. Sullivan was a brilliant and original theorist and the author of a theory of personality that is second only to Freud's in its elegance and comprehensiveness. He was also an intuitive and brilliant, if acerbic, clinician. And though he was a central figure in the turn from a nonparticipant to a coparticipant clinical paradigm of analytic work, he de-emphasized working in the transference or countertransference, of dealing directly with the immediate analytic encounter. Though Sullivan was clearly aware of transferential phenomena, he nonetheless focused on extratransference in his analyses and did not implement the coparticipatory implications of his seminal interpersonal concept of inquiry in his practice. Sullivan did not go beyond participant-observation.

Unlike Sullivan, Fromm placed great therapeutic value on immediate experience, direct engagement, and personal confrontation. Ironically enough, however, despite his emphasis on immediate experience and on direct engagement in the analytic situation (Fromm, Suzuki, and DeMartino 1960), Fromm also tended to focus on extratransference or genetic inquiry in his analytic work (Wolstein 1981c; Lesser 1992). Moreover, for both Fromm and Sullivan, participant-observation or observant participation was a one-way, authoritarian process. The analyst in this model of therapy remained the authority, the confronter, or interpreter. This was participant-observation and not yet a truly, bidirectional coparticipant inquiry, in which the patient's confrontation of the analyst would be given its just due.

The radical implications of Fromm's ideas on personal confrontation and direct contact in the analytic encounter were developed only by later generations of interpersonal theorists (cf. Held-Weiss 1984). Although neither Fromm nor Sullivan developed the full implications of their clinical ideas on the interpersonal field, both of these seminal interpersonalists contributed profoundly to the shaping of the ultimately more comprehensive concepts of coparticipant analysis practiced by later generations of interpersonal analysts.

Interpersonal analysts of our contemporary coparticipant era have inherited a dual tradition: Fromm's experiential sensibility and focus on individuation and Sullivan's operational sensibility and focus on interpersonal vulnerability (cf. preface). Fromm was one of the analysts who brought to interpersonal psychoanalysis the concept of the personal self and the importance of clinically encountering proactive individuality. This personalist focus is complemented and enriched by Sullivan's concept of an *interpersonal self* and his clinical focus on the communal aspect of human development. Whereas Sullivan's participant-observer's primary concern was the clinical management of the anxious vicissitudes of the interpersonal self in its search for safety, Fromm's humanistic, experientially oriented observant participant emphasizes the expressive uses of the personal self in the quest for self-fulfillment. The analytic implications of the contrasting foci of these two seminal theorists have been developed in the various types of coparticipant inquiry.

Contemporary interpersonal analysts, by and large, fit into one of four categories: the *traditional interpersonalists* or *classical Sullivanians*, those whose approach to treatment follows Sullivan's focus on the "detailed inquiry" and on patients' narrative reports of their extratransference experience. Second, the *radical preservationists*, like Sullivan, focus on the interpersonal self and its vicissitudes, but they have extended Sullivan's participant-observer model into a new coparticipant emphasis on here-and-now transference-countertransference transactions as co-created coparticipation. Thus, these analysts focus on the dynamic interplay of patient and analyst within the analytic field, and they emphasize a more relativist epistemology than classical interpersonalism. Third, the *radical empiricists* or *experientialists*, like the radical preservationists, focus on the intersubjectively created transference-countertransference field, but they have expanded upon Sullivanian theory with personalist and humanistic ideas and sensibilities. Concepts of coparticipant inquiry inform the work of both the radical preservationists and the radical empiricists. However, in contrast to radical preservationists, radical empiricists emphasize the curative role of immediate experience rather than that of formulative hermeneutics, and they bring a clinical focus to bear on the intrapersonal—on what I call the personal self (Fiscalini 1990, 1991) and what Wolstein (1987, 1983a,b) calls the first-personal or psychic center of the interpersonal self. Fourth, the *eclectic integrationists* or *relationists* have attempted to build theoretical and clinical bridges between ego psychology, object-relations theory, self-psychology, and traditional and modern interpersonal theory in an effort to integrate these related approaches (see, for example, the work of Greenberg and Mitchell 1983; Mitchell 1988, 1997, 2000). Most of these analysts practice some variant of participant-observation or coparticipant inquiry. Unlike traditional interpersonalists, radical preservationists and radical empiricists are characterized by their use of coparticipant forms of inquiry, including coparticipant concepts of mutual analysis, unconscious analytic communication, and shared analytic authority and responsibility. Traditional preservationists, on the other hand, tend to practice a neoclassical Sullivanian form of participant-observation or Frommian form of observant participation. Despite their many differences interpersonal analysts share a common clinical emphasis on the interpersonal self and on the field properties of the analytic situation. All interpersonalists, though they apply the field principle in different ways, highlight the interactive and intersubjective nature of the analytic process.

Coparticipant inquiry is built upon a set of participatory principles similar in several respects to those of participant-observation. Nevertheless, coparticipant inquiry differs from participant-observation in significant ways. These differences are briefly outlined in the following schematic:

Coparticipant Inquiry Relative to Participant-Observation

1. allows for greater analytic mutuality
2. provides a greater sense of copartnership
3. seeks a radical pluralism of method and metapsychology
4. is more radical in technique—including greater self-disclosure and self-expression
5. shows greater *openness to singularity* and is more open to analytic spontaneity and improvisation
6. emphasizes transference-countertransference, "here and now" analysis
7. focuses on personal self (unique individuality) as well as the interpersonal self (communal similarity)

8. encourages analysis of the analyst in the analysis

9. is less authoritarian; the analyst is not the sole authority

10. places greater focus on immediate experience and naturalness of analytic relatedness

These then are some of the major ways in which *coparticipant inquiry* has come to differ from *participant-observation*.[3]

RADICAL COPARTICIPATION: THE SEMINAL CONCEPTS OF BENJAMIN WOLSTEIN

As a form of interpersonal inquiry, coparticipation is most comprehensively developed in the work of Benjamin Wolstein (1959, 1983a,b, 1985, 1988), who coined the term to describe his conception of the analytic process as a fully interpersonal, two-way, psychological inquiry into unconscious and preconscious experience. As Wolstein points out, the analyst is not only a *participant-observer*, but also, inevitably, an *observed participant*. In other words, patients are inevitably participant observers as well as observed participants—they are *coanalysts*, whether or not they are personally, interpersonally (dyadically), or institutionally (technically) constrained from living this out in any particular analysis. This coparticipant concept of shared inquiry acknowledges patients' uniquely individual analytic resources and proclivities and allows for a radical individuation of metapsychologies and methodologies.

Coparticipant psychoanalytic inquiry draws upon the inner resources of the coinquiring patient and analyst. In contrast to other models of participant inquiry, coparticipation, as articulated and practiced by Wolstein, radically emphasizes that patients and analysts shoulder a shared responsibility for analyzing their interpersonal relations and that each bears the final responsibility for his or her psychoanalytic development.

According to Wolstein, in a fully coparticipatory interpersonal inquiry the clinical analysis of interlocking parataxes (transference and countertransference) of patient and analyst—what Wolstein (1959) refers to as transference-countertransference interlocks—may originate with either the patient or the analyst, depending on who is most capable of initiating or sustaining such inquiry at any given moment. From this coparticipatory perspective, patients' analysis of their analysts' countertransference in the immediate field of its clinical origin is welcomed as a natural expression of analytic curiosity and imagination—an expression, that is, of patients' psychological capacities for experiencing and understanding their own and their analysts' interlocking interpersonal relations.

Like Wolstein, many contemporary interpersonal analysts, particularly those I have called radical preservationists and radical empiricists, regard transference and countertransference as mutually created processes. Wolstein views every analytic dyad as generating its own unique transference-countertransference matrix. In his central concept of the psychic center of the self, Wolstein (1987) articulated the central position of unique individuality in his theory of human relatedness. In Wolstein's perspective, this individuality inevitably manifests itself in an analytic pluralism of interpretive myth and metaphor. At the same time, Wolstein emphasized the curative importance of direct, immediate analytic experience. In accordance with his radical coparticipant perspective and egalitarian principles, Wolstein maintained that the analytic situation is governed by the symmetry and mutuality of the (continuous) flow of psychic influence between its coparticipants. In other words, from the beginning of an analysis to its end, the analyst's psyche is uniquely and symmetrically present in the psychoanalytic process with that of his or her patient.

In the course of nearly fifty years, Wolstein contributed significantly, albeit almost secretly, to a radical restructuring of psychoanalytic therapy. As the contemporary Freudian Owen Renik (2000) observes,

> Wolstein was way ahead of his time. . . . His radical insistence that the implications of the uniqueness of every patient, of every analyst, and therefore of every analytic encounter be recognized makes him seem to me cutting-edge, even now. (pp. 251-252)

Renik adds:

> Wolstein's conception reminds me of the most far-reaching implications of Lacan's dictum that every psychoanalyst must reinvent psychoanalysis for himself or herself. What comes through . . . is Wolstein's clinical courage, his readiness for adventurous, honest participation within the setting of the analytic encounter; and that attitude points toward a truly collaborative clinical analytic method. In this regard, I believe, Wolstein was already heading in a direction that contemporary analysts have only just begun to explore. (p. 252)

Wolstein also contributed significantly to reshaping narrow relational conceptions of the self. Like all post-Sullivanian interpersonal analysts, Wolstein inherited a "looking-glass" model of social selfhood. Rejecting this narrow picture of humans as wholly reactive beings, Wolstein proposed a new, enlarged picture of the human psyche as fundamentally proactive in nature. This perspective on human nature informs Wolstein's concept of the psychic center of the self, which designates the inborn, individual psychological point of origin of all experience and action. Wolstein's writings convey a passionate emphasis on the centrality of psychic realism and the unique individual self. In accordance with his "post-relational" viewpoint, Wolstein abandoned the traditional psychoanalytic preoccupation with metapsychological speculation for the empirical study of the psychology of immediate relatedness and its coparticipant therapy.

Wolstein's seminal psychoanalytic vision of the personal self and its coparticipant therapy finds expression in his delineation of the therapeutic implications of individual, or first-personal, "I" processes. Wolstein advocated a new, freer form of analytic inquiry that stands in sharp contrast to the authoritarian canons of traditional psychoanalysis. Steeped in the egalitarian and pragmatic philosophy of the American school of interpersonal psychoanalysis, Wolstein proposed a democratic concept of therapeutic inquiry in which analyst and patient are coparticipant partners, capable, to varying degrees, of mutual analysis. Thus, Wolstein proposed that countertransference, like transference, could be analyzed in the immediate field of its origin, by either analyst or patient.

This radically open approach, unprecedented in psychoanalysis (except for the work of Ferenczi), argues against the traditional concern with a mythical standard technique and criticizes the restrictiveness of classical technique and its requirement of analytic anonymity, neutrality, abstinence, and the induction of regression. By contrast, coparticipant inquiry calls for analytic openness, self-disclosure, spontaneity of interaction, and the coexamination of immediate "here-and-now" experience.

COPARTICIPANT INQUIRY AND THE RELATIONAL UMBRELLA: COPARTICIPATION IN A BROADER CONTEXT

The American school of interpersonal relations has been fertile ground for the development of coparticipant concepts of psychoanalysis. Other schools have also contributed to the development of coparticipant inquiry. Especially prominent in this regard is the British object-relations school, which bears significant similarities to its American counterpart. The theories and therapies of Winnicott, Fairbairn, Guntrip, Balint, and Klein are in many ways congruent with those of Sullivan, Fromm, Thompson, Singer, and Schachtel.

The *interpersonal turn* in psychoanalysis began in the 1920s and continues to the present day on both sides of the Atlantic. Though given great impetus by the work of the American school, it also has reflected the evolving work of the British school(s) as well as that of European ego analysts.

The broad, paradigmatic shift brought about by the interpersonal turn in psychoanalysis has led to what Wolstein identifies as the ego-interpersonal paradigm in psychoanalytic practice and thought. Wolstein hypothesizes that it stands midway between an earlier biological id paradigm and the emergent post-relational psychic model of today and tomorrow. The ego-interpersonal paradigm essentially represents that perspective in psycho-analysis in which concepts of participant-observation are predominant.

In recent years, however, some modern Freudian analysts and contemporary British object-relations analysts have incorporated coparticipant concepts in their practice. These analysts have pursued more of the coparticipant possibilities of the analytic situation than the more classically oriented analysts who preceded them. For example, some modern object-relations analysts, among them such seminal British theorists as Winnicott (1947, 1958, 1965), Fairbairn (1952, 1958), Guntrip (1961, 1969, 1971), and Klein (1948, 1975), hypothesize about the many ways patients and analysts may psychologically intersect and interact with each other. For example, they often make use of Klein's concept of projective identification in theorizing about the analytic relationship between patient and analyst and the complex ways in which they deeply and unconsciously impact on one another. Racker's (1968) work on countertransference and transference also bespeaks a coparticipant sensibility: analysis seen as a field phenomenon and the patient seen as a real copartner with a greater analytic role. This is not coparticipant inquiry at its most radical or comprehensive, but it points in that direction. Contemporary object-relations theorists, such as Thomas Ogden, Neville Symington, and Christopher Bollas, by and large practice relatively conservative variants of coparticipant inquiry; their approach is more conservative than that followed by many modern American interpersonalists, as seen, for example, in the work of Edgar Levenson, Arthur Feiner, and the late Benjamin Wolstein.

Some contemporary Freudian analysts have also developed an interactive concept of the psychoanalytic situation and greater appreciation of the transactional nature of the patient-analyst relationship, as can be seen, for example, in the following comments by Abrams (1992) on the psychoanalytic process:

> While the process can be conceptualized as what goes on *within* the mind of the patient, those steps can only be set in motion by the interaction *between* the participants. Analysts treat people, not minds. The analyst-patient relationship is a partnership with a defined approach designed to achieve a goal too difficult to define with precision at first. (p. 76)

Abrams clearly shows a coparticipant sensibility. However, many contemporary Freudian analysts tend to be relatively conservative in their analytic approach and basically follow a liberalized nonparticipant model of psychoanalytic praxis, despite their incorporation of a more interpersonalized, concept of analytic relatedness. Some modern Freudians, however, do practice a variant of coparticipant inquiry. Such contemporary Freudians as Theodore Jacobs and Owen Renik practice in ways that include coparticipant concepts of inquiry.

Conservative coparticipant trends in British object-relations and modern Freudian psychoanalysis are mirrored in the post-Kohutian work of such intersubjective analysts as Robert Stolorow, Donna Orange, Howard Bacal, and George Atwood. These modern theorists practice intersubjective psychoanalysis based on their interpersonal orientation, and they employ an analytic methodology and approach derived from concepts of a Heideggerian phenomenology and Gadamerian hermeneutics mixed with the self-psychological concepts of Heinz Kohut (cf. Stolorow, Brandchaft, and Atwood 1987; Stolorow and Atwood 1992; Stolorow, Atwood, and Brandchaft 1994).

Kohut's psychology of the self, a late contributor to the evolving interpersonal turn in psychoanalysis, is focused on the same dimension of the personality that the American interpersonal theorist Sullivan had emphasized—the analytic vicissitudes of the interpersonal self, the inherent human need for interpersonal security and social approval (see chapters 6–9 for a critique of Kohut and self-psychology). Despite this theoretical complementarity, self-psychological analysis and interpersonal therapy diverge greatly (see chapter 8 for a detailed critique of Kohutian praxis). For example, interpersonal analysis follows a much bolder form of coparticipant clinical inquiry than self-psychology, which essentially has remained tied to classical or neoclassical conceptions of the analytic process. Though Kohut advocated an interpersonal or object-relational metapsychology, his technique was still orthodox Freudian, even though self-psychology brought a radically new stance of prescribed empathy to the analytic task. The concept of prescription runs counter to the improvisatory sensibility of coparticipant inquiry. In comparison with the radical coparticipant inquiry of the American school, Kohut's coparticipant perspective is relatively conservative. However, Kohut's modern day successors, self-defined intersubjectivist theorists, follow a more interactive concept of analytic inquiry that rivals that of the American school.

Intersubjectivity theory, like contemporary interpersonal theory, holds a coparticipant notion of transference and countertransference as born in interaction and shaped jointly. Stolorow and his collaborators (Stolorow, Brandchaft, and Atwood 1987; Stolorow, Atwood, and Brandchaft 1994) focus on the analytic interactivity of analysts' and patients' subjectivity. Their contextual view of the analytic situation as an intersubjective experiential field evidences a coparticipant sensibility that is, in some ways, radical (for example, their theoretical emphasis on a relativistic and constructivistic post-Cartesian epistemology). Yet, clinically, their work, like that of object-relations theorists, represents a relatively conservative form of coparticipant inquiry. For example, there is no call for a bolder, freer, or radically expressive technique; their analytic method remains largely neo-classical Freudian, with its strict reserve and formality. There is only a limited sense of true analytic copartnership or of a methodological (or metapsychological) pluralism. In sum, reliance on coparticipatory inquiry is limited.

Given their emphasis on the centrality of contextual analysis, inter-subjectivists focus one-sidedly on the analysis of the interpersonal, reactive self—the self as appraised and defined by others (one's self-objects). Implicitly, they de-emphasize working with the personal self, that is, the self-subject or proactive self. Thus intersubjectivists, like interpersonal radical preservationists, limit their coparticipatory inquiry to the inter-personal or intersubjective dimensions of their patients' psychology, leaving aside their important personal and subjective dimensions—their patients (and their own) unique individuality. These latter factors are, in fact, what provide the conceptual foundation for the most comprehensive and radically oriented variants of coparticipant inquiry.

The situation is somewhat similar for modern Freudians with a coparticipant sensibility, such as Owen Renik, Ted Jacobs, and the late Merton Gill, who constitute the leading edge of contemporary Freudian approaches to psychoanalytic praxis. Renik (1993, 2000) showed himself to have coparticipant inclinations in his study of the continuous mutual engagement of patient and analyst, and Jacobs (1991, 1995, 1998) and Gill (1982a,b, 1983) also leaned in the same direction in their respective interpersonal focus on the interactive analysis of transference and countertransference. Renik's coparticipatory sensibility is also evident when he writes movingly of the critical importance of personal freedom and authentic individuality for both patient and analyst:

> More and more, I find myself thinking that the essence of the clinical analytic enterprise involves the patient being able to identify his or her personal freedom and use it. It hasn't been my impression that received psychoanalytic wisdom has encouraged analysts to identify and use their personal freedom. Our field has not developed in a way that facilitates the courage—if I can put it that way—of individual analysts. All too often, our elders have subtly advocated conformity of one kind or another. (2000, p. 253)

Despite increasing evidence of a growing coparticipant sensibility in mainstream psychoanalysis, contemporary Freudian analysts—much like intersubjectivists and contemporary object-relations theorists—practice a form of coparticipant inquiry that remains relatively limited. For example, in a discussion of self-disclosure in psychoanalytic work, Jacobs takes what I consider a very cautious, deliberate, conservative stance. In particular, he believes "that there is often—most often—very good reason for the analyst not to disclose his [or her] thoughts or feelings to the patient" (1995, p. 239).

Though developments in post-Freudian psychoanalysis move toward coparticipant inquiry, currently they are still largely less egalitarian in spirit and less free in technique and therapeutic coparticipant initiatives than the more radical practice of analysts of the American interpersonal school.

The differences between current developments in coparticipant inquiry and the various neoclassical versions of the neutral, silent, nondirective mirror analyst are striking. Although many versions of post-Freudian technique have grown considerably more liberal, more dyadic in concept, and more human in tone, they nonetheless still represent a conservative, relatively reserved and restrictive technique, and a general monadic sensibility.

Inasmuch as the various object-relations approaches to the psychoanalytic situation also draw from the coparticipant model of praxis, there is a significant overlap between these approaches and contemporary interpersonal perspectives on coparticipant inquiry. Many of the characteristic features of coparticipant analysis are also implemented in the work of modern object-relations analysts. Nevertheless, these approaches tend to be more conservative in technique, more authoritarian in concept, less open-ended, less pluralistic, and less radical in their field orientation, and more preoccupied with matters of metapsychology than those analysts who consistently and comprehensively practice in more radical coparticipant terms.

The more comprehensive use of coparticipant concepts in the clinical approaches of contemporary interpersonal analysts such as Edgar Levenson and the late Benjamin Wolstein is based on an understanding of the analytic situation as a human encounter, an experiential field in which the analytic process is jointly shaped by the two participants. This dyadic process is characterized by mutuality and reciprocity. Patient and analyst are seen as *copartners* whose relationship is democratic and nonhierarchical. Both coparticipants are free to choose their preferred methodology and metapsychology. The coparticipant orientation also emphasizes immediate experience, acknowledges each individual's uniqueness, and gives greater priority to patients' psychology than to analysts' metapsychology.

In addition to focusing on the vicissitudes of the interpersonal self, coparticipant inquiry, in contrast to participant-observation, attends to the critical analysis of the personal self. This dimension of the work is essential because the most radical forms of coparticipant inquiry, the most truly two-way coparticipant processes, require a concept of a personal self, or unique individuality.

In recent years, relational psychoanalysis, which is practiced by those modern Freudians, self-psychologists, interpersonal relations analysts, intersubjective analysts, and British object-relations analysts who follow some form of participant-observation or coparticipant inquiry, has gained wide popularity. This rubric covers a complex array of theoretical and clinical approaches that share a two-person clinical sensibility and a common emphasis on the primacy of psychosocial or interpersonal factors in the formation and functioning of personality and of fantasy (intrapsychic) experience. The various relational schools emphasize the interactive and intersubjective nature of the psychoanalytic process. Analysts who identify themselves as relational vary in how radical or conservative they are in their coparticipant approach to psychoanalytic inquiry.

The relational school is not a school with a single specific theory and clinical practice, for it is essentially a school of schools, with all the diversity that implies. Unlike the traditionally recognized psychoanalytic school that evolved out of a seminal figure's creative vision, relational theory refers to a collection of related schools. It is, in other words, a metaschool and thus represents a meta-metapsychology. Analysts often identify themselves as relationists for various pragmatic or political reasons, as, for example, looking to legitimize, justify, or reserve the right to freely borrow from several psychoanalytic traditions or to create a hybrid form of psychoanalytic thought and practice. Of course, what this metaschool gains in generality it loses in specificity and singularity. It does not represent nor propose a new, unique vision of human nature nor a new version of *homo psychoanalyticus* nor a new, creative vision of psychoanalytic praxis. Instead, it gives political weight and theoretical legitimacy to the social philosophies and clinical concepts of the seminal figures of the various broadly relational schools; in this way it provides a needed counterbalance to the historical exclusiveness of Freudian analytic orthodoxy.

Recent efforts to draw distinctions between relational theory and interpersonal theory (cf. Hirsch 1998; Frankel 1998) are ultimately a forced and fruitless task, for these theories exist on different, incommensurate levels of abstraction. Comparing interpersonal theory and relational theory is like comparing an apple with fruit or a horse with animals or a Chevrolet with cars. Interpersonal theory is subsumed under relational theory, an individual instance of a more general category.

However, the various schools sheltered under the relational umbrella can be compared with one another. The more radical nature of the interpersonal varieties of coparticipant inquiry, as contrasted with the more conservative coparticipant practices of the other schools of the relational umbrella (self-psychology, object-relations, ego-psychology, and intersubjective analysis) is clear from the following list:

Characteristics of Radical vs. Conservative Coparticipant Inquiry

1. greater self-expressiveness of therapeutic experience; freer expression of spontaneous thought or feeling;

2. more self-disclosure of feelings or biographical fact;

3. greater focus on immediate experience, rather than formulative hermeneutics;

4. more focused on the relationship, rather than interpretation, as agent of therapeutic change. Focus on curative instrumentality of living through processes;

5. conceptions of origin and nature of transference and countertransference are similar, but there is a greater focus on the analysis of countertransference in the analytic session itself;

6. less concern with "proper" analytic stance or the "frame;"

7. more egalitarian and less authoritarian;

8. greater openness to a pluralism of metapsychologies;

9. more active confrontation of patients' defenses; there is a striving for an optimal balance of comforting and confronting;

10. advice more freely given and freer use of what classical theory calls "parameters";

11. much greater focus on self-fulfillment, the personal self, and unique individuality;

12. greater working acknowledgment that there is no one "right way" or "right answer." There is a greater focus on a pluralism of interpretive formulations and procedural methodologies. This is based on the notion of the uniqueness of each analytic dyad.

13. greater focus on personal agency and personal responsibility.[4]

Coparticipant inquiry is the emerging model of psychoanalytic praxis today. Rooted in the interpersonal sensibility and radical experiments of Ferenczi and the interpersonal concepts of a more relational, interactional ego-psychology, object-relations theory, and self-psychology, it is informed by contemporary developments in interpersonal psychoanalysis.

Coparticipant inquiry is practiced in both conservative and more radical ways. In turn, radical coparticipant inquiry divides into what may be called the *relational* and the *experiential* modes of coparticipation. Relational coparticipation is marked in interpersonal theory by concepts of radical preservation and the transformable analyst as well as by a focus on the interpersonal self. In contrast, experiential coparticipation is characterized in interpersonal theory by radical empiricism, an existential sensibility, and a focus on the life of the personal self.

Coparticipant inquiry, whether of the relational or experiential variety, builds upon and stands in contrast to participant-observation (traditional Sullivanian inquiry) and observant participation (traditional Frommian inquiry) as well as nonparticipant mirror-observation (classical Freudian technique). In its experiential mode, coparticipant inquiry is exemplified in the clinical work of a number of contemporary interpersonal and relational psychoanalysts, who, like Ferenczi and Freud long before them, look to find new and more alive ways to explore the ways of the human psyche.

Let's now turn to a study of the multidimensional self and its dialectics, in particular, its experiential dimensions, dynamic functions, and the therapeutic implications for coparticipant inquiry.

PART TWO

THE SELF

CHAPTER 4

The Multidimensional Self

Coparticipant inquiry is premised, in part, upon a unique vision of the self. For the inquiring coparticipant psychoanalyst the notion of the self—the "I" or "me"—is a compelling study, critical to the understanding of human experience and behavior. Yet questions of the true nature of the self remain. Is it a unitary phenomenon or multidimensional in nature? Inborn or acquired? And, if learned, how? Are we inviolably separate from one another, or are we all in some fundamental sense indivisible, transpersonally linked. Or, paradoxically and beyond logic, are we somehow both: indivisibly connected, part of a unity, yet profoundly separate?

The psychoanalytic study of the self and the answers to questions such as these has been an open project, reflecting evolving and differing conceptions of human nature. From Freud's ego and Jung's actualizing self to Laing's divided self and Wolstein's psychic center of the self, the various psychoanalytic traditions have offered diverse visions of human selfhood and its development and dynamics. These different perspectives on the self have had significant implications for the various psychoanalytic theories of clinical engagement and therapeutic process.

The psychological concept of the self comprises a complex family of psychic processes and experiences that have been defined and conceptualized in many different ways. With the possible exception of its close theoretical relative, the concept of narcissism, the self is arguably the most variably defined concept in contemporary psychoanalytic theory. Nevertheless, it is deemed theoretically relevant to almost every aspect of psychoanalytic thought and practice, and it is perhaps the most critical conceptual lens now in use in psychoanalysis. Used in such different ways by different theorists, the term *self* has acquired a multitude of conflicting and sometimes confusing usages, invested with a broad range of meanings.

In ordinary discourse, the self refers to individual persons and all they experience as "belonging" to themselves—their body, psychological self, etc. This meaning of the self extends to include all that people define as "mine": from relatives and family, personal attachments and social memberships, material possessions, and creations to states of mind, emotional life, desires, or motivational dispositions.

This broad and common-sense definition of the self, *self-as-person*, thus encompasses the individual person and all of his or her qualities of being and having—the totality of "I," "me," and "mine." Those in the psychological sciences, however, define the self in narrower terms as *self-as-personality*, limited to the person as a psychological being. In an even more limited fashion, the self is often variously defined by psychologists as self-as-social role or self-as-psychic process (*self-as-agent*). More commonly, it is defined reflexively as *self-as-representation*, or self-personification, what some call self-as-object, or simply self-image or self-concept.

This definitional diversity, in which the same term is used variously to refer to one or more different psychic processes or experiences, is further complicated by inconsistencies in terminology; the same term is used to refer to different aspects of the self and different terms (such as the "ego" or "I") to refer to the same aspect of the self. Thus, for example, what the theorist of the self Carl Rogers (1951, 1961) refers to as the *self* (i.e., self-concept or self-as-object), other psychological theorists may call the *ego*. Conversely, those functions that many theorists label as belonging to the ego, others define in terms of the self. Generally, however, those processes of the self that are seen in terms of as self-as-agent are designated as proactive parts of the ego or the "I," whereas those that form parts of the self-concept or self-image are referred to as reflexive aspects of the self or "me." Confusing things further, some theorists use either term, self or ego, to refer to either or both of these aspects.

Critical of this confusion, the noted personality theorist Gordon Allport suggested the use of the Latin term the *proprium* to refer to those aspects of individuality that we ordinarily call the self. Within this rubric Allport (1955) comprehensively identified eight self, or propriate, functions: bodily sense, sense of self-identity, ego-enhancement, ego-extension, self-image, the rational coper, propriate striving, and the cognitive knower, what James (1890) called the pure ego.

Within this broad definitional context those who study the self psychologically or psychoanalytically tend to divide the self into two different forms or aspects: the self-as-proactive-process or self-as-subject and the self-as-reflected appraisal, that is, the self as made up of the opinions and evaluations of others. This reflexive self-as-object comprises what I call the *interpersonal self*, the socially defined self—in James's term, the "social self" or what we could call the other-in-the-self. In contrast, the self-as-proactive process refers to that broad set of processes and potentials in the self that I call the *personal self*. This includes that innately given set of psychological potentialities and traits that define the self-fulfilling and self-realizing capacities of the individual. The personal self includes aspects of James's spiritual self and pure ego.

This division of the self into self-as-subject and self-as-object reflects a central controversy in the psychoanalytic theory of the self—whether the psychic self is socially or individually constructed and developed. Is the self an individual given or a social construction? This central question has been answered in various ways by different personality and psychoanalytic theorists who have focused on different aspects, functions, and dimensions of those phenomena we collectively call the self.

Foremost among psychological theorists who have focused on the study of the self is William James, whose lengthy and comprehensive chapter on the self in his 1890 *Principles of Psychology* still stands as a classic treatise on the subject. A generation later, James's fellow American, the renowned psychiatrist and interpersonal theorist Harry Stack Sullivan developed his own theory of the reflexive self; he was influenced by James's pragmatic philosophy and democratic spirit as well as by the American thinker, Charles H. Cooley and his looking-glass concept of the self. Sullivan was also inspired by the American social philosopher George Mead and his view of the reflexive self as socially constructed. Sullivan's theory of the self is arguably the most theoretically sophisticated, extensively researched, and clinically relevant psychoanalytic theory of the self, with the possible exception of Karen Horney's cultural-interpersonal formulations. Sullivan certainly contributed the most extensive and detailed study of the self as an interpersonal phenomenon to psychoanalysis.

Sullivan's field perspective on the self as emergent communal experience is, in my estimate, the psychoanalytic theory of the self that is most compatible with a coparticipant theory of psychoanalytic inquiry. Coparticipant inquiry implicitly requires a notion of human selfness that considers the human being an inherently and irreducibly social being. Sullivan's concept of the self and its dynamic relation to interpersonal anxiety fits this requirement perfectly, as will be discussed shortly when I consider the interpersonal self. However, this only satisfies half of the theoretical equation, for coparticipant inquiry requires a dialectical, complementary notion of an individual or personal self—a concept of the irreducible human striving to fulfill or realize one's unique psychic promise. This promise did not find a place in Sullivan's theory; however, a broader psychoanalytic theory of the self, incorporating a concept of a personal self, can be advanced that is compatible with Sullivan's interpersonal focus. This notion of unique personal individuality taken together with Sullivan's interpersonal focus forms a broad theoretical foundation for coparticipant inquiry that is premised on a dialectical view of the human psyche as being simultaneously social and individual, neither dimension of this duality being reducible to the other.

THE INTERPERSONAL SELF

Sullivan viewed the self as a social product, as born in interaction with others, shaped by the inherent human need to avoid anxiety. The self encompasses all that living that is known to consciousness as well as the vast system of unconscious defensive processes or security operations that keep the phenomenal or personified self intact and unchanged.

This extensive system of reflexive psychic processes and defensive, self-protective patterns constitutes the domain of the interpersonal self. This concept of the self's activity based on interpersonal relations and reflexive social process makes Sullivan's schema of the self a natural theoretical underpinning for coparticipant inquiry.

The self, in Sullivan's words, represents the "sum of reflected appraisals" (1940, p. 22) of oneself by the significant others in one's development. The self is an interpersonal process, learned, developed, and ultimately known only through one's living among others. True to his vision of mankind as inherently and irreducibly communal, Sullivan focused on the adaptive, reactive, and consensual in human experience.

The interpersonal self forms a necessary theoretical foundation for a coparticipant psychoanalytic inquiry, but it is insufficient because it does not explain will, agency, intention, and other self-active or proactive processes that are essential for coparticipant therapeutic inquiry.[1] Nevertheless, the concept of an interpersonal self, socially constructed and defined, addresses a clinical truth and analytic reality—the absolutely critical clinical role of self-esteem and its analytic vicissitudes. Sullivan, like Kohut many years later, knew firsthand the almost overwhelming clinical importance of the domain of the interpersonal self or social selfhood.[2]

According to Sullivan's version of the interpersonal self, the self is defined or bounded by the need to free itself from anxiety. For Sullivan, anxiety defines a family of dysphoric emotions; in its more primitive forms it is the intense experience of "awe, horror, dread, or loathing" (1953, p. 10).

In Sullivan's view, the self and anxiety are dynamic reciprocals. The self is made up of all conscious experience that is speakable or thinkable (i.e., socially approved and not too anxiety-provoking to admit into consciousness). Anxiety, like the interpersonal self it creates and circumscribes, represents a fundamental process in human psychopathology as well as a pivotal dynamic in analytic inquiry.

According to Sullivan, personifications, or representations, of oneself and others, apprehended initially in rudimentary form as primitive patterns of interpersonal experience with *good mother* and *bad mother* and involving *good me, bad me*, and that personal evil, the uncanny and terrifying dissociated *not me*, are developed under the necessity to discriminate experience (reflected appraisals) so as to avoid or minimize disapproval and gain approval. Originally, "caught," induced empathically, from significant mothering others, anxiety, becomes the parameter that defines awareness; and the self-system, the ever-watchful guardian of self-esteem and acceptable consciousness, forms that "vast system of processes, states of alertness, symbols and signs of warning" (Sullivan 1954, p. 101) that comprises the anti-anxiety dynamism.

Self-esteem and approval mean the same thing, the human imperative that Sullivan called the need for interpersonal security. He believed all human beings inherently have the need to feel safe and secure in the presence of others. To be insecure is to be anxious, and the anxiety of disapproval or "loss of love" originates from that disapproval *itself*. For Freud, however, the anxiety of loss of love (or of any other hypothesized danger situation, e.g., castration, ostracism) derives from the danger that this loss of approval or love brings—the trauma of helplessness in the face of overwhelming biological excitation. Thus, in Freud's system the need for interpersonal security is secondary, not primary and is derived from its relation to the relief of instinctual tension. Anxiety is the human (and also animal) reaction to potential sensory overload. In Sullivan's system the need for interpersonal security is primary and not derivative. One simply *needs* to be secure with others, not because to be so *means* relief of a physiological drive.

In Freudian theory anxiety derives ultimately from human powerlessness, the inability to stop the flood of sensory excitation. For Sullivan, it is not powerlessness itself but the experience of it as inadequacy that leads to anxiety. Powerlessness in itself leads to fear rather than anxiety. Interestingly, Sullivan initially viewed power (in the sense of capacity or ability) as an important aspect of the need for security. Later, however, he revised this conception, limiting the concept of power to that of a neurotic security operation (i.e., the effort to control or dominate others, what Fromm [1947] calls the attempt to exercise power *over* others). I will consider Sullivan's theory of the power motive further when I address the possibility of a more expansive psychoanalytic theory of the self.

It is important to note that such terms as anxiety, insecurity, disapproval, or low self-esteem are pale terms for the humiliating, terrifying, and nightmarish experiences they refer to. Similarly, such terms as security, approval, or freedom from anxiety do not readily convey the intense, thrilling, or calming and even beatific emotional quality of feeling adored, cherished, loved, and valued. It is a sad fact that few among us, whether patient or analyst, experience such positive or even euphoric states of wholeness and worthiness consistently. Psychological maturity does not merely signify the capacity for doing one's duty and being loyal, responsible, and generally grown-up. It also refers to an aliveness of thinking, richness and depth of feeling, and spontaneity of relatedness. Sadly, this is not a state that many in our society attain. As Sullivan trenchantly observed, from the pernicious effects of anxiety and the creation of limited and limiting personified selves, all too often people become caricatures of *what they could be*. However, in what we could be, what we can become, lies hope for us all.

It could be argued, as May (1953) does, that Sullivan's interpersonal concept of the self and anxiety represents a cultural or personal bias and that the need for interpersonal security and self-esteem represents a particular personal or cultural concern rather than a universal human imperative. While the experience of anxiety is universal, it is a matter of conjecture whether its origins are interpersonal. Sullivan's exclusive concern with the realm of the interpersonal self and his relative neglect of the personal self may reflect the narrowing effect of historical or cultural influences. Nevertheless, I am convinced that Sullivan mapped a crucial dimension of the human psyche. Perhaps more than any other theorist, he studied and elaborated its clinical and therapeutic significance.

Important as the clinical study of the interpersonal self is, a more complete and fuller study of the strivings of the individual can be achieved by considering some aspects of the self that Sullivan ignored or only touched upon marginally. These processes form a psychic dimension that may be included as an integral part of an expanded and more comprehensive psychoanalytic theory of human motivation and the self. Though the interpersonal self is doubtless a central dimension of human experience and crucial in the coparticipant analysis of the psychopathology of the self, other processes of the self also need to be studied for a comprehensive coparticipant account of the human psyche.

OTHER DIMENSIONS OF THE COPARTICIPATORY SELF

Sullivan's theoretical system assumes three basic groups of human needs and three types of threats to the self if these needs are unmet. Security, as already noted, is freedom from anxiety, and satisfaction refers to the gratification of bodily needs, including the genital drive. The third group is the need for interpersonal intimacy, that very important set of relational needs that begin in infancy as a "need for contact" and develop into a need for intimacy and love. Unmet need for love is loneliness, a motive thought by many to be an even more powerful motive than interpersonal security.

A comprehensive and multidimensional theory of the self emerges when two additional important groups of selfhood are included in the psychoanalytic theory of the self. These processes are implicit in several of Sullivan's conceptions and in the conceptions of some theorists of other schools, but neither they nor Sullivan have attended to these specific processes in any systematic way. They are explored in the theoretical work of some interpersonalist theorists of a humanistic and existential (experiential) bent, most prominently by Fromm (1947, 1955, 1964), Fromm-Reichmann (1959), May (1953, 1967), Schachtel (1959), Singer (1965), Wolstein (1981a,b,d, 1983a,b, 1987), and, more recently, Fiscalini (1990, 1991, 1994a,b), Wilner (1998a,b, 1999), and Frie (1999, 2001, 2003).

These two additional sets of motives and sources of self-experience I call (1) *the personal self*, or the need for self-fulfillment, for freedom from *dread*, the fear of psychic death or self-constriction; and (2) *the personalized self*, the need for personal orientation and organization, for freedom from *apprehension*, the fear of novelty, uncertainty and disorganization.

Before moving on to a discussion of dread and apprehension (i.e., the personal and personalized selves) and their clinical significance for coparticipant inquiry, I would like to note very briefly those aspects of selfic experience I call the relational self and the physical, or sensual, self.[3]

THE PHYSICAL SELF

This dimension of the coparticipant self includes the vast set of psychosomatic processes involved in the human striving for physiological, sensual, or biological satisfaction, ranging from the basic needs for life: oxygen, sleep, food, water and freedom from injury, pain, or harm to one's physical integrity and health, through the span of sensual needs collectively referred to as lust or sexuality to the manifold of kinesthetic and myriad other sensory phenomena and processes of motility of all sorts.

Traditionally, orthodox psychoanalysts have focused on the sexual aspect of this dimension of the self. Sexuality represents a central human motive and is an important aspect of most analyses. Nevertheless, many contemporary Freudians are increasingly informed by interpersonal and relational concepts and no longer consider sexuality the central or exclusive focus of clinical inquiry.

The striving for bodily satisfaction is implicated in all that goes on in an analytic inquiry. Still, in my estimate, this dimension of the self does not carry the analytic significance of the psychic domain of the interpersonal self or the personal self. For instance, lust only takes on clinical significance when seen in dynamic relation to the interpersonal self, that is, when lust becomes suffused or interpenetrated with concerns about social acceptability and shame, guilt, or anxiety. In fact, lust only becomes a psychiatric or psychoanalytic problem when it meets with internalized social disapproval. Nevertheless, sexuality is a frequent enough topic of coparticipatory exploration. As Sullivan (1953, p. 203) points out, lust, the "felt component of the genital drive," is a major motivational system. Sullivan hypothesizes that lust is a human need that emerges only later in development, usually not until puberty. He maintains, however, that once "lust gets under way, it is extremely powerful. In fact, if one overlooks his experience with loneliness, he may well think that lust is the most powerful dynamism in interpersonal relations" (p. 266). Sullivan emphasizes that lust is a major source of anxiety and conflict, at least in our culture, which he regards as "the most sex-ridden people on the face of the globe" (p. 289).[4] An extensive and comprehensive study of the physical, or sensual, self and its relations to the interpersonal, relational, and personal selves is a study worthy to pursue but must wait for another day.

THE RELATIONAL SELF

The relational self refers to that broad set of purely interpersonal or social needs that express the innate human striving for contact with others. The relational self, in other words, defines a complex set of interpersonal motivations, encompassing, in Fairbairn's (1952) term, the object-seeking dimension of human personality.

This cluster of interpersonal needs is expressed in the many ways in which humans strive for verbal and nonverbal communication. The relational self, then, includes all those primary needs for interpersonal attachment, affiliation, affection, engagement, responsiveness, and intimacy that are met in interpersonal experiences such as empathy, sympathy, attunement, affective interplay, participant play, emotional connectedness or resonance, being known or knowing, seeing and being seen, parallel play, companionship, friendship, love, and similar forms of interpersonal sharing. The component aspects of the relational self may be ordered developmentally, ranging from early, primitive and often one-sided forms of intimacy to the more mature states of intimacy, which in their higher forms are characterized by the experience of mature love and full mutuality.

Developmental observations (cf. Schecter 1973; Stern 1985) indicate that infants and young children search for intimate interpersonal experience, even if in developmentally primitive ways. Sullivan (1953), too, recognized the need for intimacy as a need that is inborn or acquired early. And he recognized its developmental structure and outlined a theory of it. Although Sullivan explored the later developments of the need for intimacy, he did not elaborate its early expressions in infancy and childhood. Sullivan's theoretical effort, as noted earlier, was focused on elaborating his theory of the interpersonal self and anxiety, rather than on formulating a developmental theory of intimacy and the relational self.

The developmental structure of interpersonal intimacy remains an aspect of contemporary psychoanalytic theory that requires further detailed study. The work of developmental theorists such as Schecter (1973, 1978) and, more recently, Stern (1985) and Beebe and her collaborators (Beebe and Lachmann 1988; Beebe and Jaffe 1997), are significant steps in this direction. In fact, the findings of Stern, who has a definite interpersonal sensibility even though he doesn't define himself in those terms, have been revolutionary, turning most psychoanalytic theories of the origins of the self on their head. Stern's research suggests that the young infant does not, as has been conventionally thought, start out in a blind, selfless symbiotic tie to others. Instead, already quite early on, infants bring a more self-aware sense of themselves to sought-after interactions with their mothering figures.

Interestingly, the seminal interpersonalists Sullivan and Fromm, like many developmental theorists of other analytic schools, have tended to underestimate the young child's relational capacities for mutuality and love. Sullivan, for example, asserts that intimacy does not emerge until preadolescence. I think this is open to question; the capacity for love seems to emerge much earlier. Although the capacity for intimacy may not mature or come to full fruition until preadolescent development or even later (or, unfortunately for many people, never), it seems to exist, albeit in limited form, much earlier. Young children often appear capable of what seems like genuine empathy and sympathy.

Children may exhibit submissive or symbiotic forms of "love," but this is a defensive expression of the interpersonal self, not of the relational self; it is a matter of security, not intimacy. Though both are interpersonal in nature, the relational self and the interpersonal self refer to very different dimensions of self-experience and self-process.

To summarize: The relational self is based on the need for interpersonal intimacy, on the inherent human need for engagement, affection, and mutuality. By contrast, the interpersonal self is based on the human need for interpersonal security, for social approval, status, prestige, and the like. And though love and approval may be closely related and are often mistaken for one another, they are not the same.

THE PERSONAL SELF

Although the interpersonal self represents a central dimension of coparticipant inquiry, it is too narrow a concept to fully encompass a comprehensive and multidimensional understanding of coparticipant analysis. A corrective to this theoretical limitation lies in the recognition of the psychological domain of the personal self. A full appreciation of the radical possibilities of coparticipant inquiry requires a concept of those creative and proactive psychic processes and potentialities that I call the personal self. The dynamics of the personal self comprise that set of psychic processes, motives, and experiences that are marked by the human striving for self-realization and self-expression.

The personal self may be defined as the innate and immediate proactive striving of the self to live out one's singular psychological capacities or unique individuality. It includes the drive to develop and express one's originality—one's own psychological powers and capacities, personal and interpersonal—in all fields of human experience.

The personal self defines the *personal source of all psychological action—feeling, thinking, imagining, wishing, willing. It is the self-moving originator of psychic experience.* It is the source of creativity, spontaneity, play, and those processes we call will—intending, determining, choosing, initiating. It is the *source of psychic agency.* The personal self encompasses both one's active, organizing self—the processes that organize mental representation and behavioral activity—and one's proactive, creative self—all those processes involved in the striving for self-fulfillment.

The group of processes I call the personal self comprises the psychic analogue of the need for bodily satisfaction. It refers to what Wolstein (1981a,b) calls psychic self-fulfillment, and it overlaps with aspects of those human existential needs that Fromm (1955) terms sense of identity and transcendence. The need for fulfillment refers to the innate human striving for personal expansion and self-knowledge and the fulfillment of one's unique psychic potential, including the full expression and realization of one's capacities for feeling, imagining, and thinking. Fromm (1955) termed this aspect of selfness the active center of the self, what Wolstein (1983a,b) called the "I" or first-personal, unique self, and Winnicott (1958) and others called the true self. In one sense, the personal self is akin to the relational self, to the need for interpersonal intimacy; however, here the need is for self-intimacy, the need to know and to be oneself.

Frustration of fulfillment is inevitable for everyone though its extent is always individual. The dread of unfulfillment, of unlived life, may be experienced as longings to "be fully oneself," wistful yearning for something more, feelings of emptiness, or a vague sense of wanting. It may also be experienced as anxiety, fear, or even loneliness. Severe or prolonged dread of unfulfillment, what Fromm-Reichmann (1959) has aptly referred to as psychological death, may lead ultimately to resignation or other states of apathy, often accompanied by repressed rage and hostility.

The processes that comprise the personal self are explored in the theoretical work of some contemporary interpersonalists. The personal self is recognized in the humanistic thrust of the work of Leslie Farber (1966), Rollo May (1967), and Erwin Singer (1965) and also in Clara Thompson's (1958) notion of an inherent tendency to develop and grow, and Frieda Fromm-Reichmann's (1959) and Karen Horney's (1950) explicit discussions of an innate dynamic of self-realization. Moreover, Erich Fromm's (1947, 1955) ideas on individuality and self-realization and Benjamin Wolstein's (1981a,b, 1983a,b) extensive and detailed studies of "I" or first-personal processes, unique individuality, and psychic self-fulfillment point in the same direction. Many analysts of other schools of psychoanalytic thought and practice have also studied this dimension of the psyche. This is especially true of those who integrate concepts of existential analysis into their clinical practice (cf. May 1967; Frie 2003).[5] Sullivan's focus on the interpersonal aspects of living, in terms of the relational self and the interpersonal self, precluded a full appreciation of the singularly personal and the self-actualizing domain of the self.

Sullivan's positivistic emphasis on operationalism led him to focus on what could be observed in consensus and to eschew what he termed the delusion of unique individuality. Wolstein's (1959, 1977) post-Sullivanian perspective on unique individuality and his extensive study of its therapeutic role has done much to correct Sullivan's neglect of this critical psychological dimension. In a scholarly critique of Sullivan's view of operationalism, More (1984) argued convincingly that Sullivan's application of the physicist Percy Bridgman's operational methodology was unduly restrictive and that analytic consideration of unique individuality does not violate standards of scientific operational study—that, in fact, science always includes the private and individually unique.

A contemporary psychoanalytic theory of the self that incorporates the clinical relevance of *both* the interpersonal and personal selves provides a foundation for the full unfolding of a truly coparticipant psychoanalytic inquiry, one that is both interpersonal and deeply personal.

THE PERSONALIZED SELF

The dread of unused or unlived psychic life conflicts with the fear of freedom and new experience that I call apprehension. This basic human fear of the unfamiliar or inchoate underlies the set of human motives and processes I call the personalized self, the need for personal orientation and organization, or freedom from apprehension.

The personalized self includes the human needs for order, coherence, familiarity, certainty, and predictability, and it includes aspects of those existential needs that Fromm (1955) calls rootedness and frame of orientation and devotion. When this need remains unmet, apprehension results. Apprehension includes what Kierkegaard poetically refers to as the dizziness of freedom and what Schachtel (1959) calls embeddedness anxiety and what others describe as a fear of the unknown, unfamiliar, or ambiguous.

Sullivan touches upon the dynamic of apprehension when he talks about the fear of novelty. He also refers to the human need for familiarity and predictability when he speaks of the reassuring power of language to label the otherwise nameless or, in a more sardonic vein, of man's "evil genius for rationalization." But he did not elaborate these ideas into a theory of apprehension. Sullivan's theory of resistance, however, addresses a crucial aspect of the need for personal orientation. According to Sullivan's theorem of escape, the self-system, the defensive anti-anxiety dynamism, "from its nature . . . tends to escape influence by experience which is incongruous with its current organization and functional activity" (1953, p. 190).

In other words, we all tend to perpetuate our ways of being and experiencing—to seek familiar structure. In this way, people fail to profit from their experiences and thus compulsively and futilely repeat neurotic patterns. Sullivan implicitly accounts for this not only in terms of the specific interpersonal anxiety that any particular change in the self-system occasions but also, and very importantly, in terms of the anxiety or fear that is aroused by reorganization of the self-system or a characterological shift This is what I call apprehension. Thompson (1950) refers to it as secondary anxiety. In other words, it is not simply the old danger, the original threat to the self that is the problem; there is a new source of danger, the disorganization or reorganization of the personalized self, of the personified "me" or representational self. *Apprehension, thus, is the fear of change itself.* The threat to the self emanates from new, as yet unknown selfness. Apprehension thus is the fear of new experience, rather than bad experience. As Thompson (1950) puts it, the threat of

> change to . . . the nature of the self-system is all that is needed to produce anxiety. . . . By the time the self-system is formed, there is an emotional stake in maintaining it blindly and this forms a rigidity in the personality and increases the potentiality for anxiety. (p. 126)

Schachtel (1959) addresses the same issue even more emphatically:

> man is afraid that without the support of his accustomed attitudes, perspective, and labels he will fall into an abyss or flounder in the pathless. . . . Letting go of every kind of clinging opens the fullest view on the object. But it is the very letting go which often arouses the greatest amount of anxiety. (p. 195)

Thus, for Schachtel, anxiety is essentially fear of separation from the known; it is the fear of personal disorientation or loss of structure that I call apprehension. Schachtel's theory of anxiety, like Schecter's (1973), was deeply influenced by Fromm's conceptions of anxiety that were, in turn, deeply influenced by those of Freud. In fact, Fromm's theory of anxiety may be understood as a cultural-interpersonal-existentialist translation of Freud's biological concept of separation anxiety. Although their anxiety theories differ in metapsychological emphasis and detail, Freud, Fromm, Schachtel, and Schecter all share a concept of anxiety based on separation, and in this they differ from Sullivan. Both Schachtel (1959) and Schecter (1973) explicitly reframe Sullivan's interpersonal concept of anxiety (and its hypothesized empathic mode of transmission) in terms of separation, that is, as a special case of separation or stranger anxiety. I disagree and don't think that either anxiety or apprehension can be reduced to the other; they are separate and distinct forms of threat to the self and describe different, though dynamically related, dimensions of the self.

THE MULTIDIMENSIONAL SELF: A SCHEMATIC

The multidimensionality of the psychoanalytic self and its dialectic of the personal and the interpersonal forms the theoretical premise for coparticipant inquiry. Coparticipant analysis demands a concept of the strivings of the self I call the personal self (the need for self-fulfillment) and those opposed needs for security that I call the interpersonal self.

All analyses, coparticipant or not, are characterized by the conscious and unconscious interplay of the five dimensions of the self. Phenomenologically, these various dimensions of the self often resemble one another. For example, the tensions of apprehension and dread—the blockage of the personalized and personal selves—are phenomenologically similar to those experiential states we call anxiety, fear, or loneliness. Apprehension is subjectively similar to fear, and the pattern of tension that ranges from yearning or emptiness to dread has components of both loneliness and fear. Both apprehension and dread, however, usually lack the qualities of shame, humiliation, or sense of self-loathing that often give complicated interpersonal anxiety its characteristic experiential stamp.

Table 4.1 Dimensions of the Coparticipant Self

Self Dimension	Need	Self-Threat
Physical self	Satisfaction	Fear
Relational self	Intimacy	Loneliness
Interpersonal self (representational self)	Security	Anxiety
Personalized self (representational self)	Orientation and organization	Apprehension
Personal or authentic self (self as agent)	Fulfillment	Dread

These five dimensions of the self and self-threat to the self can be schematically represented as shown in table 4.1.

In the psychoanalytic situation, the five dimensions of the self all intersect and interact, and most analytic behavior and experience results from the simultaneous operation and influence of two or more self dimensions.[6] These interactions and their clinical implications will be examined next in chapter 5. But first we'll take a brief look at motivational theory and the multidimensionality of the self.

MULTIDIMENSIONALITY OF THE SELF AND MOTIVATIONAL THEORY

Motivational theory in psychoanalysis has drawn from two models of the human being, the regressive and the progressive. The regressive model of human motivation sees individuals as striving for release from accumulated tension, for a regressive return to an earlier state of presumed quiescence, of little or no stimulation or arousal. This view of humankind is represented most unambivalently in Freud's formulations of libido and mortido as exemplified in his constancy and Nirvana principles. It has been similarly represented in psychology by the tension-reduction perspective of Hullian behaviorism. In contrast, the progressive model of motivation sees humans as primarily striving for activity and seeking stimuli (Singer 1965). The individual is seen as striving for optimal sensory arousal rather than sensory quietude; excitation and stimulation are sought rather than avoided. The progressive view is represented, for example, in Gardner Murphy's (1958) yen to discovery, Jerome Bruner's (1966) will to learn, and Robert White's (1959) concepts of effectance and neurogenic drive. The empirical findings of psychologists such as Robert White, Harry Harlow, and Robert Berlyne (cf. White 1959; Singer 1965; Fromm 1973; Eagle 1984) clearly indicate that humans have fundamental drives to explore, investigate, manipulate, and, in Goldstein's (1939) phrase, come to terms with their environment (and themselves). This work confirms the progressive view that phenomena such as curiosity and wonderment are primary and inborn, and not simply sexual, relational, or interpersonal derivatives.

According to the progressive view of human motivation, shared by humanistic personality theorists and by the major heterodox psychoanalytic theorists, the individual is essentially forward-moving and inherently seeks to expand or realize himself or herself. This view of mankind posits a self-actualization or self-fulfilling dynamic as a major motivational principle. Personality theorists who posit a self-actualizing dynamic either regard it as a kind of master motive, a superordinate tendency that defines all of a person's strivings, or, like Abraham Maslow (1967), they view it as one among other human motives. This latter point of view then allows for a plurality of motives and a model of human beings as having both regressive and progressive tendencies.

In contrast to the more delimited concept of tension-induction, the concept of self-actualization is an extremely broad psychological construct. As such, it has been criticized as being too general and vague a concept, as unscientific, metaphysical, or even mystical. The concept of self-actualization is, in fact, difficult to define or measure in precise, operationally testable, terms (and this may account in part for Sullivan's disinclination to advance such a concept). Maslow's (1971) answer is that we need different, holistic-analytic, concepts of science. In any event, whatever its conceptual or epistemological limitations (cf. Eagle 1984), the concept of self-actualization seems to have an intuitive, almost self-evident, quality of truth. Although we may differ considerably in our definitions of human potentiality, I think we all intuitively sense that there is some inherent human striving to fulfill ourselves, to actualize our potentials, or to make real our deepest capacities and desires.

For self-actualization theorists who posit this dynamic as the single superordinate human motive, the concept runs the danger of being reductive. In this sense, self-actualization theory becomes as reductive as Freud's sexual drive theory or Sullivan's interpersonal theory. Everything, all motivation, becomes reduced to the single unitary motivational principle, whether it be psychic self-actualization or sexual homeostasis or, if one is a reductive interpersonalist, social homeostasis. Like Freud's pleasure principle (or, more broadly, the principle of hedonism), the principle of self-actualization can be stretched to cover all the data, even those that seem to contradict it. When used to explain everything, the concept explains nothing and becomes empirically irrefutable or, in Popper's (1965, 1968) term, unfalsifiable.

Theorists who posit pluralistic, rather than unitary, concepts of motivation and the self avoid this criticism, but they may engender their own set of problems. Maslow (1971) is perhaps the theorist best known for integrating the dynamic of self-actualization within a pluralistic motivational theory, one that recognizes a multiplicity of motives.

There is some similarity between my motivational categories and those of Maslow (1971). We differ markedly, however, in our views as to the relations among these different motives. Maslow orders his motives hierarchically, with physiological needs at the bottom of his motivational pyramid and those of self-actualization at the top. And he regards the lower needs as motivationally of higher priority, with higher needs only attaining motivational force when the lower ones are satisfied. I cannot agree with this view and have not ordered my motivational schema hierarchically. Instead, in my view all motives are expressed from the very beginning, and priority is determined by interpersonal experience, not by any a priori ordering. Which motive has priority at any given moment is determined in a complex interaction and cannot be predicted. Speculatively, I would suggest that personal fulfillment is the strongest of all motives and not, as Maslow suggests, the weakest. On the other hand, his concept of fulfillment (self-actualization) is a narrower construct than mine.

In the next chapter I will examine the clinical features and interactive dynamics of the dimensions of the personal, interpersonal, relational, physical, and personalized selves. In particular, I will focus on the dynamic relation between the strivings of the personal self and the opposing tensions of the personalized self and the interpersonal self. The implications of this dialectic for coparticipant analytic inquiry will also be explored.

CHAPTER 5

Clinical Dialectics of the Self

The human psyche is characterized by a fundamental dialectic between its communal and its uniquely individual dimensions, between its strivings for social adaptation and for self-fulfillment and self-expression. The psyche is at once reactive to its social environment and also personally proactive; it seeks interpersonal security as well as personal creativity. This dialectical nature of the psyche is manifest in the dynamic relation between the interpersonal and personal selves and in the dialectic of the other selves: the personalized, relational, and sensual selves.

The personal self, as defined earlier (cf. chapter 4), comprises processes of will, autonomy, agency, and creativity, among other aspects of unique individuality. It thus represents the subject side of the psyche. Though it may be developmentally influenced by interpersonal experience—its various aspects affirmed or disconfirmed, approved or disapproved, prescribed or proscribed—its core is inviolably personal and private, uniquely individual and nonrelational. In other words, the personal self cannot be reduced to the interpersonal or relational selves anymore than they can be reduced to it. Human beings are inherently social yet also uniquely individual. A full account of the human psyche thus requires a balanced consideration of both dimensions of the self (as well as of those of the relational, sensual, and personalized selves).

Historically, psychoanalytic attempts to understand our paradoxical psychological nature—of being both consensually interpersonal and uniquely individual—have often resulted in efforts to resolve this paradox by reducing one psychic dimension to the other. Rather than view the psyche in paradoxical terms, analytic theorists have preferred to simplify things through reductionism. Either the uniquely individual in some way is seen as interpersonally derived or the interpersonal is reduced to the individual. Yet the paradoxical nature of our psyche remains. Though involved in nearly constant interaction with others (either intrapsychically or interpsychically), living out our desires for contact with others, we are also inevitably alone, living out our desires for creative solitude. Man's individuality cannot be reduced to the social, as Sullivan and other interpersonal and object-relational theorists would have it, and the social cannot be reduced to the individual (and biological) as Freud and orthodox analysts would have it. Our inborn psychological potentials and proclivities interact with our social surroundings from the first moments of life. We exist from the very beginning within a social field, but we are not reducible to that field.

In the coparticipant clinical situation, there is a continuous dynamic tension and dialectic between our needs for fulfillment, satisfaction, and love and our limiting or conservative needs for personal orientation and interpersonal security. All of these needs may coexist and operate simultaneously in any particular experience or psychological action. Moreover, any one of them may appear defensively as any one of the others.

Clinically, disentangling the motivational influences of the various dimensions of the self can be a complex analytic task. Consider, for example, a common and relatively simple situation where an individual's striving for self-fulfillment is frustrated, as when a patient is unable to freely live out an aspect of his or her creativity. Is this patient's blocked self-realization a reflection of interpersonal anxiety, of the dynamic play of the interpersonal self, or of apprehension, that is, the fear of the unknown? In what ways is it perhaps a mix of the two? And does fear play a role? What are the sources of a particular patient's subjective sense of urgency about his or her lack of demonstrated creativity? Is this a matter of interpersonal anxiety? Narcissism unfulfilled? Or perhaps a situation in which the individual's self-regard, prestige, or sense of self-acceptance depends on being regarded as special and creative. Some other anxious dynamic? Or is it a question of dread, psychic constriction, or suffocation? Or is at the root perhaps a complex amalgam of dread and anxiety?

Similar complexities characterize the relationships among all five sets of the self's needs and the threats to the self they occasion when not met. Depending on the particular situation and individual, one or another of these sources of threats to the self may get priority in terms of motivation. For example, when an individual frankly criticizes a friend, openly expresses a so-called "perverse" sexual desire, speaks out in defense of an unpopular idea, or publicly supports a politically incorrect position, these behaviors, depending on their interpersonal context and personal meaning, may predominantly reflect the play of the personal self or the interpersonal self. They may signify processes of spontaneity, assertiveness, and personal authenticity and integrity (the personal self) or a defensive dynamic based on impulsivity and hostility (the interpersonal self). Clarifying the psychic role and interplay of the various dimensions of the self in these and other behaviors is, in my view, best achieved through a coparticipant analytic inquiry into the patient's extratransference and transference relatedness. In this process the patient and analyst, working coparticipantly, jointly attempt to separate out the impulsive from the spontaneous, the defensive from the self-actualizing.

It is particularly difficult to differentiate the clinical play of the relational and interpersonal selves. Clinical expressions of the relational and interpersonal selves often are ambiguous; it is often hard to tell which one is clinically operative in a particular therapeutic or life situation. This may be due to the fact that both refer to the same social side of the self even though to different dimensions of it. For instance, a patient may cry bitterly in telling of a loved one's coldness, emotional distance, or lack of empathy and affection. It may be difficult for analyst and patient, even with extended inquiry, to ascertain whether this clinical behavior reflects relational grief and loneliness or interpersonal impotent rage, whether it springs from a threatened interpersonal self—from a defensive dependency and anxiety about aloneness—or arises from an unmet relational self—from love unrequited. Most likely both dimensions of the self are at play; however, it can be difficult to sharply delineate the ways in which they are dynamically intertwined in their transference and extratransference aspects.

The relational and the interpersonal selves overlap in significant ways even though they represent different psychic aims. For example, true approval of another (the interpersonal self) always engenders a love for them (the relational self). And love for another always opens the self to acceptance of this other. There is no question that those who feel unaccepted also feel unloved. The relational and interpersonal selves are most difficult to differentiate in their developmentally more primitive forms, in which the search for intimacy and that for security are often complexly intertwined. It is in these early states of the relational and interpersonal selves that they clinically most resemble one other. For example, a patient's wish for empathic resonance is often a complex expression of the wish for love and for security. Another example is the situation of "falling in love." When does the delight, the headiness, and the sexual passion of a newly found mutual love represent a mutual narcissism, a found self-object experience, a defensive infatuation—the clinical expression of the interpersonal self, of anxiety and the need for security? And when does it reflect the emergence of the relational self, of a desire for intimacy, for relational attachment, a breaking down of previous barriers to intimate connection? For example, a patient, a young married woman in her early thirties, strives futilely to have her authoritarian, old-fashioned parents recognize her and to "be known by them," to have their agreement on a number of matters and subjects. Is this a desire for intimacy and closeness? Or is the interpersonal self at work—the need to be thought worthy of being understood, the need to matter and be approved of? Of course, there are many questions here. Why, for instance, does the patient, at this point in her life, still need her parents' recognition? Furthermore, how does this all play out analytically? These and many other therapeutically relevant questions will form an integral aspect of a coparticipant psychoanalytic inquiry into the patient's psychic difficulties. Nevertheless, it is often difficult to differentiate the clinically similar, but dynamically different, manifestations of the relational and interpersonal selves.

In my view, the clinical complexities and dialectics of the various dynamics in the self are best explored in a coparticipant inquiry that fully recognizes the uniquely individual analytic capacities and proclivities of the coparticipant patient (and analyst).

It may be observed that just as powerlessness to meet vital biological needs leads to fear, so psychic unfulfillment, the powerlessness to meet vital psychic needs, leads to dread. Thompson's (1950) notion of an inherent "tendency to develop and grow" and Sullivan's concept of a drive to mental health both imply that the human striving for fulfillment of one's psychic capacities or resources may be stronger, or prove stronger, than anxiety. Is dread really more powerful than anxiety? Is the human need to fulfill oneself stronger than the need for the approval of others? What happens when strivings for fulfillment are thwarted? It is difficult, or perhaps impossible, to determine an answer in the abstract since there is great individual variation. Some individuals strive to realize their uniqueness, even under conditions of severe anxiety and apprehension. For others, security rules, and self-realization recedes. In fact, humanistically inclined psychoanalytic theorists such as Rollo May and Erich Fromm, among others, complain that the individual of today out of fear has opted for social conformity rather than for individual creativity. Obviously, one's interpersonal history is crucial. There are significant differences in the degree to which individuation, creativity, and self-expression are encouraged or discouraged in any particular historical time, culture, or system of family practices. Nevertheless, however truncated or inhibited the need for self-fulfillment may become, it is always there. And it is in these self-strivings and the self's capacities, in dealing with the dread and moving toward a personal self, that we find our ability to move through our fears, apprehensions, and anxieties.

CLINICAL ASPECTS OF THE PERSONAL SELF

In the psychoanalytic situation, when the analyst is open to this psychic dimension in the patient, he or she may hear dread or strivings for personal fulfillment, where previously only manifestations of anxiety, loneliness, or fear were heard (cf. Fiscalini 1990). What from the perspective of interpersonal security may seem like psychopathology, defensiveness, or even almost autistic behavior may from the perspective of unfulfilled dread appear as idiosyncratic, or even eccentric, moves toward self-realization, whether lived out in relationships or only privately. Although the patient's efforts to achieve his or her full selfness are not inherently interpersonal, they are conditioned by the interpersonal, and they eventually express themselves within a shared context, namely, in the social field of psychoanalytic therapy (as well as in the social fields of everyday life).

The analyst may discern the patient's strivings for self-fulfillment as they emerge and express themselves in dynamics such as personal insight and other steps toward self-knowledge, new thoughts and original formulations or perceptions of oneself and others, developing abilities to bear anxiety, apprehension, guilt, sadness, grief, disappointment, frustration, and other distressing emotions and experiences. Other indications of the patient's movement toward self-fulfillment are his or her increasing capacity to be alone in the presence of the analyst, curiosity about the analyst and the analytic interaction, engagement in countertransference analysis and analysis of the analyst's counterresistance, various idiosyncratic moves toward personal growth even if they look like resistance, and making changes in one's life.

Dread develops whenever anxiety and apprehension prevail in an individual's approach to a situation. If not worked through, this dread, or thwarted fulfillment, leads to impotent rage and ultimately to depression and even physical death. This can take the form of the slow death of conventionality and neurotic adaptability (what might be called the neurosis of normality). Dread is revealed in wistful longings for achievements of one sort or another, in wishes to make a mark and do something meaningful with one's life. Of course, these wishes may be mixed with adolescent or infantile drives for glory, competitive victory, or other defensive evasions of anxiety or apprehension. Patients may also express fears that they can't achieve some important goal of self-fulfillment and engage in self-protective efforts to restore self-esteem. This may be accompanied by feelings of irritability and rage and even depression, and it may give rise to various addictive or compulsive ways of trying to cope with and compensate for pervasive feelings of inner constriction, hollowness, or deadness.

The need for self-fulfillment is a human imperative. Of course, it is possible that what I think is universal and fundamental simply reflects a personal or cultural bias. After all, what I call dread could simply be anxiety about irrationality or helplessness, interpersonally conditioned. Such anxiety may always be mixed in with dread, but I do not think that dread is reducible to interpersonal anxiety. It is a primary and significant source of personal terror. The yearning for self-fulfillment, the potential for dread, runs deep in us all. Psychoanalysts who have explored this aspect of the psyche have addressed a central dimension of human living, one that finds only marginal recognition in the interpersonal, object-relational, and self-psychological study of anxiety, which is focused on the interpersonal dimension of experience.

Like the majority of other interpersonalists, Sullivan, given his operationalist views, did not attend to the dimension of self-threat I call dread. However, his coevals, the prominent interpersonal theorists Clara Thompson and Frieda Fromm-Reichmann both acknowledge this dimension of the psyche. Fromm-Reichmann (1959) addressed the phenomenon of dread in her hypothesis that psychic stagnation represents an important source of anxiety. Fromm-Reichmann thought that the futile repetition of parataxic or neurotic interpersonal patterns—i.e., the inability to change—leads to a fear of "psychological death" analogous to the fear of physical death and forms the basis of many people's anxiety. Though Fromm-Reichmann did not distinguish this anxiety from interpersonal anxiety in Sullivan's narrower sense of the term, she nonetheless points to a source of tensions resembling anxiety that is not necessarily interpersonal.

The experience of dread, however, is generated not only by the dissociated repetition of futile interpersonal patterns of relatedness but also by other ways in which the human need for self-fulfillment may become inhibited or impaired. For example, Thompson points to the "anxiety" of dread in her observation that "any threat to the expression of one's potentialities is anxiety producing" (1950, p. 129).

The broadening of psychoanalytic theory to include a self-actualizing dynamic has clinical as well as theoretical implications. First of all, it contributes to a greater and more explicit appreciation of patients' therapeutic needs for affirmation of their strivings to actualize their psychic potential. Such relational interventions may be technically intended and explicit, but they often happen implicitly and unconsciously in that inadvertent form of therapeutic relatedness that defines the *living through* process, which underlies the working through process (Fiscalini 1988; see also chapter 3). This sort of experience may account in part for certain unexpected therapeutic successes that would otherwise seem improbable given the patient's apparent unfavorable therapeutic attitude (e.g., a limited receptivity to interpretive insight). The inadvertent affirmation of the patient's self-actualizing needs may occur even when the analyst consciously dismisses or eschews the notion of a self-actualizing dynamic. In such instances, the analyst implicitly holds a self-actualizing concept of the psyche though in a deeply private way. In such cases, the analyst may ascribe therapeutic progress to other, actually irrelevant, analytic factors.

The explicit inclusion of a self-actualizing motive in psychoanalytic theory expands the range of clinical interpretation in the coparticipant psychoanalytic situation. As noted earlier, when open to this dimension of the patient's psyche, the coparticipant analyst will see the patient's behavior differently, and at times he or she will hear the strivings of the personal self for fulfillment where he or she previously may have heard only the signs of anxiety or loneliness, that is, the strivings of the interpersonal and relational selves. What may seem like defensiveness, resistance, or neurotic pathology from the perspective of interpersonal security may be understood as individual moves toward individuation, autonomy, personal growth, self-expression, and self-realization from the perspective of personal fulfillment. With a more attuned interpretive ear, the coparticipant analyst may discern previously unrecognized self-actualizing themes in the patients' narrative reports as well as in their interactive coparticipation in the analytic dyad.

Consider, for example, the following: an analyst returns from a brief family holiday. Her patient is very curious about the analyst's family vacation and asks questions about it. The patient, married and with children herself, has exhibited a similar passionate curiosity on a few other, seemingly unrelated, occasions. It is not new behavior but relatively rare. The curiosity has an intrusive and insistent tone, which suggests a defensive dynamic, but at the same time it has an alive quality to it. How are we to understand the patient's curiosity? A separation anxiety? Hostile envy? As a defensive sexual derivative, perhaps a strongly activated primal curiosity? Or is it a controlling wish to know secrets about the analyst? Perhaps it represents a wish to know how the analyst enjoys herself and relates to her family on such occasions so the patient can model her own behavior; the analyst knows that the patient tends to be symbiotic and overly dependent and looks to others to tell her how to live. Or is it all a defensive evasion of some other, more anxious, analytic topic? These and other defensive uses of the patient's curiosity are all possible, and on the basis of previous work some seem probable.

However, if we shift from the perspective of interpersonal security, or self-protective defensiveness, we can also view the patient's behavior from the standpoint of a drive toward relational intimacy, a wish to know about the analyst, and to know who the analyst is. Perhaps the intrusive and insistent quality bespeaks a defensive fear that the patient's transferential love for the analyst will not be accepted. Is her curiosity an essentially timid, albeit defensively aggressive, form of love? A bid for closeness? The analyst (perhaps relaxed by her vacation) is uncharacteristically more relaxed and open in answering several of the patient's questions. Has the patient, emboldened by the analyst's openness, become more open herself, freer than usual, momentarily less inhibited in asking the questions she has yearned to ask? Is the patient seeking a transferential intimacy, a relational closeness, rather than acting in a distancing and defensive resistance?

The analyst is concerned that she is abetting a defensive curiosity on the part of the patient and wonders about her possible countertransferential collusion in this. But is the analyst's countertransference of a different nature—is it, instead, her inhibition in answering questions on previous occasions? Has the analyst, in fact, been involved in a chronic transference-countertransference replay of a parental dampening of the patient's childhood aliveness and capacity to wonder? The analyst notes her own previous incuriosity about the patient's experience of curiosity, of the patient's relationship to her imagination. The analyst notes, with a sharpened awareness, the patient's general tendency to be incurious about her and her living situation. The patient's fear of using her own psychic resources is experienced by the analyst with a vividness previously unfelt. The analyst becomes more curious about the patient's curiosity and its defensive and self-striving aspects. Why is the patient generally not curious about her and her analytic participation? Has she simply been inhibiting her curiosity, fearful of expressing it? What are the conditions of her curiosity? What frees (or inhibits) this capacity and its expression? Perhaps the badgering tone of the patient's questioning hides a deeper and truer curiosity.

The patient's curiosity, in other words, is now seen as more than an instrumentality in the service of interpersonal security, relational intimacy, or sensual satisfaction. It can also be understood as the expression of a deep desire to fulfill her personal capacity for wonder. Now the analyst has not only matters of anxiety and loneliness (or fear) to consider but also matters of dread—of the natural history of this patient's frightened relationship to her own gift for wondering. In other words, the patient's interaction with the analyst can be examined as a dynamic of fulfillment as well as one of security or intimacy (or satisfaction). Of course, the therapeutic understanding of the patient's curiosity does not come from the analyst alone but arises out of the patient's and analyst's imaginative coparticipant inquiry into their intersecting experiences.

The coparticipant analyst may also discern patients' strivings for self-fulfillment and individuation in various emotional or symptomatic expressions of dread and, as previously noted, in such analytic behaviors as the direct coparticipant analysis of countertransference, counterresistance, and counteranxiety (as well as transference and resistance analysis). Other indications for such strivings are spontaneous analytic relatedness, moves toward self-knowledge, "new" thoughts, and imaginative or original perceptions and conceptions of the self, the analyst, the analytic interaction, and events in the larger world. The patient may also show greater analytic assertiveness and independence, as in holding to his or her own interpretations even if they conflict with those of the analyst, in developing greater sense of personal conviction about his or her intuitions, newfound abilities to bear anxiety, shame, sadness, rage, and other dysphoric experiences. Further indication of patients' individuation is seen in their self-disclosure, increased capacities to criticize as well as care for the analyst, and the ability to "surrender" to the influence of the analyst and his or her interpretations, in the sense of considering them, not simply swallowing them without thoughtful review.

An analytic awareness of the dynamics of the personal self and the need for self-fulfillment contributes to a greater sense of the patient as a copartner in the analysis. The analyst can see the patient as more resourceful and capable of collaborative and responsible coparticipatory analytic inquiry than would be predicted by psychoanalysts who hold a regressive (and authoritarian) theory of motivation. Though the ability to do analytic work is highly individual and conditioned by each patient's unique life experiences, the more progressive view of the individual as proactive, self-actualizing shaper of his or her fate allows, I think, for a generally healthier, more optimistic, and more respectful view of the patient and his or her analytic and psychic capabilities. It allows for a more open and nonauthoritarian concept of analytic inquiry.

In contrast to authoritarian prescriptive concepts of the analyst as the sole provider of interpretations and sole structurer of analytic procedure, the coparticipant approach views the patient as able, at least potentially, to do his or her full share of the analytic task. An analytic appreciation of patients' innate needs for personal fulfillment facilitates, for example, the recognition of their desires and abilities to develop or define their own personal metapsychology (which, ironically enough, may not include a self-actualization dynamic). Or, more radically, the coparticipant viewpoint is premised upon the centrality of the personal self to analysis and encourages patients and analysts to create together the analytic methodology that best suits their unique capacities and needs.

The coparticipant view of the patient also emphasizes the patient's ultimate responsibility for his or her maladaptive and unfulfilling life. Thus, in the analytic situation, the coparticipant patient is held responsible for the resistive aspects of his or her coparticipation and held capable of working productively with therapeutic confrontation of his or her neurotic desires and defenses. Consequently, the coparticipant analyst strongly encourages his or her patient to explore the personal roots of his or her anxiety, even if it makes for an uncomfortable analytic experience. In other words, the notion of a personal self fosters and supports a more direct, confrontative, and coparticipant analytic approach than is characteristic of more traditional analytic approaches to praxis. Whereas addressing the patient's interpersonal self introduces the analytic themes of interpersonal influence and vulnerability, focusing on the personal self highlights the analytic themes of personal resilience and responsibility. Coparticipant inquiry strengthens the autonomous personal self instead of merely reassuring the insecure and other-directed interpersonal self. More is asked of the patient, and the patient responds with more.

Premised on the concept of a personal self and on the clinical dialectic between this personal self and the dynamics of the interpersonal self, the coparticipant analytic approach maintains that patients carry within them the inner strength, resources, and ultimate existential freedom to find and shape their own truths and future living within the limits of their abilities and the constraints of their social environment.

ON ANXIETY AND APPREHENSION

For many analysts, particularly those of an interpersonal or object relations direction, interpersonal anxiety forms the major disjunctive force in psychic life. This view is articulated most clearly and comprehensively in the interpersonal conceptions of Sullivan (1940, 1953, 1954). Sullivan considered the crippling experience of interpersonal anxiety the source of inappropriate and inadequate interpersonal relations and the root of analytically relevant discontinuities in experience and distortions in living. In his view anxiety is centrally implicated in all that comes to analytic attention, what the practicing analyst must "eternally deal with" (1954, p. 107). In his clinical and theoretical work, Sullivan focused on the study of the interpersonal self, on the analytic play of the universal human need for security, safety, and approval. The analytic vicissitudes of interpersonal anxiety and its parataxic concomitants form the core of psychoanalytic inquiry, according to Sullivan.

Clinically, apprehension is often mixed with interpersonal anxiety. The fear of psychological change usually stems from the apprehension of the unfamiliar and the fear of aloneness and lack of approval. Apprehension, though not inherently interpersonal, is almost always conditioned by the interpersonal. Some people grow up in homes where exploring, entertaining ambiguity, and similar attitudes are encouraged. And their life reflects this background—they are strikingly unapprehensive. Other people grow up in fearful, harsh, or restrictive homes in which life is shown to be full of peril and in which venturing forth is viewed with alarm. Undoubtedly, the unknown and ambiguity will be linked with considerable anxiety and fear in such instances. When a person grows up in a home where obsessional omniscience, narcissistic grandiosity, or paranoid vigilance and fear of spontaneity are necessary defenses. Of course, none of us are ever entirely free of apprehension and anxiety. They affect us differently, depending on our individual history of interpersonal relations and our inborn individuality.

In the psychoanalytic encounter the patient has the opportunity to live out his or her apprehension and anxiety with the analyst. When not countertransferentially or counterresistantly anxious or apprehensive, coparticipant analysts may experientially (and interpretively) live through their patient's fears of fulfilling themselves directly with the patient in the living through process of the personal analytic relationship (Fiscalini 1988; see also chapter 13). There, the patient has a new and reconstructive experience with a significant other who is less afraid, apprehensive, and anxious about the patient's or his or her own individuality and psychological growth than the historically significant others in the patient's life were. When this process occurs in the analytic inquiry, therapeutic growth is greatly facilitated—one could say it becomes inevitable. Analytic self-transformation largely occurs in this experiential, emotionally corrective, and silent way.

Of course, the process of therapeutically living through anxious and apprehensive analytic experience depends on analysts' alertness to the play of apprehension and anxiety within themselves, their courage in facing this, and their awareness of the complicating effects of their own anxious past experience in venturing toward personal fulfillment. Most fundamentally, however, it depends on the analyst's own unconscious or preconscious capacities for growth and change. Openness to growth in another always implies its correlate in oneself. The analyst's functional capacity for personal growth defines the limits of his or her therapeutic availability and of the patient's therapeutic opportunity, at least in that particular analytic situation. In other words, at any given moment in analysis the dyad can only go as far as the more mature partner of the two. If the analyst's anxious complication of his or her own apprehension obscures the patient's apprehensiveness, leads the analyst to distort it as anxiety, or causes the analyst to falter in his or her capacity to follow it out analytically with the patient, then the analyst cannot be therapeutically present and will fail the patient, at least for that moment. In withdrawing from the coparticipant inquiry, at least momentarily, both analyst and patient may feel less apprehensive and less anxious. But both will also be less alive, albeit secure in their defenses.

This sort of countertransference operates silently in many analyses. As a result, many lengthy analyses, even those that have been successful in many ways, leave significant aspects of the patient's (and analyst's) pathology or characterology unresolved and untouched. In other words, when congruent or complementary transference-countertransference (or more precisely, resistance-counterresistance) patterns, resulting from similar or overlapping apprehensions and anxieties, are operative in an analysis, growth is hindered, and this often goes unnoticed by both participants. This happens in situations where the patient and analyst share personal blind spots or pathological attitudes common in their culture (as, for example, the patterns of competitiveness, controllingness, and materialistic cynicism so common in our culture). These silent transference- countertransference problems often lead to prolonged, even intractable mutual analytic dependencies, to lengthy analyses that die a slow death of boredom and result in mutually "satisfactory" conventional adaptations. They can also lead to situations in which the analysis ends and proves helpful in many ways but remains incomplete in significant ways. Sometimes the patient continues or completes his or her unfinished work in a later reanalysis, perhaps even with the same but now changed and matured analyst. Too often, however, analysts cannot provide such constructive resolution for themselves.

By limiting oneself to the familiar and organized one can avoid apprehension, but it also gives rise to the threat of psychological death, the dread that comes from stagnating in one's development for fear of venturing into new and unknown psychic territory. As Schachtel (1959, p. 45) warns, "the seeking of protection in the embeddedness of the familiar makes for stagnation and constriction of life." And this is as true for the analyst as for the patient.

ON SELF-ESTEEM AND SELF-REALIZATION: THE DIALECTIC OF THE INTERPERSONAL SELF AND THE PERSONAL SELF

Our needs for fulfillment, satisfaction, and love often conflict with those for personal orientation and interpersonal security. Our needs for creativity and self-fulfillment to some extent always oppose our need for order, stability, coherence, and the consensual approval of others. If we are to grow and fulfill our potential, we must endure the painful experiences of apprehension and anxiety. As Fromm (1955) reminds us:

We are never free from two conflicting tendencies: one to emerge from the womb . . . from bondage to freedom; another, to return to the womb, to nature, to certainty, and security. . . . Each step into . . . new human existence is frightening. It always means to give up a secure state . . . which was relatively known, for one which is new, which one has not yet mastered . . . at any new step, at any new stage of our birth, we are afraid. . . . The whole life of the individual is nothing but the process of giving birth to himself; indeed, we should be fully born, when we die—although it is the tragic fate of most individuals to die before they are born. (pp. 32–33)

In their prolific and often eloquent writings on humankind's psychological dilemmas, Fromm and May, both humanistically oriented cultural-interpersonal psychoanalysts, repeatedly point to our fears of creativity, self-expression, and individuation. Both point to our common existential plight—our ultimate aloneness, mortality, and powerlessness before nature—and to our need to create a personally meaningful relatedness to ourselves, others, and the world. Fromm and May each lament the modern individual's all too common flight from existential freedom and responsibility into addictive conformity, anxious masochism, sadistic destructiveness and compulsive competitiveness. These are the ills of unfulfillment—the psychopathology of everyday life—we see daily in our clinical work with individuals who have the hope, courage, and inner resources to attempt the arduous and painful psychoanalytic inquiry into the self and its various dimensions. But in our society most people's needs for growth and self-transformation go unheeded both by themselves and by others, at great personal and social cost.

I think May (1953, 1967) is correct in maintaining that to be psychically whole, each individual must bear his or her existential fears and apprehensions of freedom and originality (what one might call "apprehension of the creative leap") while seeking his or her own personal answers to them.

Each individual also must develop an ability to bear and analyze his or her irrational interpersonal anxieties if he or she is to grow psychologically. As analysts, we are all aware that both anxiety and apprehension move behavior in directions consistent with the limiting envelope of our interpersonal and personalized selves. As analysts know all too well, throughout the course of analysis both patient and analyst are inevitably confronted with the opposition of their defensive self-systems. Any movement toward therapeutic insight and growth invariably entails the distress and pain of both anxiety and apprehension and the defensive counterthrust of our ego defenses or security operations, as we strive self-protectively to restrict our experience to the familiar and acceptable.

It is vital for both analyst and patient to bear their own anxious and apprehensive experience and that of the other in the coparticipant analytic situation. Although, as Sullivan observes sardonically, "nobody wants anxiety," the patient must gradually learn to bear his or her anxiety and apprehension, to experience them, and work them through. Though this process may prove painful at first, the patient must develop (with the assistance of the analyst) from within his or her personal self an increasing capacity to communicate and to learn in the presence of anxiety and apprehension. This form of self-confrontation is, of necessity, achieved in small steps, and takes considerable time, but it cannot be rushed and cannot be abrupt, for sudden, intense anxiety and apprehension simply stun the self and stop analytic work.

As Sullivan (1954) cogently reminds us, the analyst should "administer no wounds that do not heal" (p. 234). An essential feature of therapeutic skill is the ability to chart a course between the Charybdis of too much anxiety and the Scylla of too little. In this in-between space the patient is able to work through and resolve his or her patterns of anxiety and apprehension and their derivative psychopathology.

In addition, as May (1967) emphasizes, the coparticipant analyst must help his or her patient to develop the capacity to bear his or her real guilt and enduring regrets. Every patient has harmed both himself or herself and others, whether they were loved or hated. It does not matter whether this harm was necessary psychologically or unconscious and done unknowingly. What matters is that we do not, in May's (1967) words, "push aside the pain or cover over the tragic possibilities" (p. 108). This holds true for the analyst as well as for the patient, and in this truth lies a strong impetus for counterresistance. This applies to our sense of having betrayed our responsibility toward others and also of having betrayed our own self-potential, of having been unfaithful to ourselves.

Ultimately, it is only through the painful and frightening, yet also liberating and joyful experiencing fully our past beings and our present becomings that we can fulfill ourselves and work through our apprehension, anxiety, and dread.

PART THREE

NARCISSISM

CHAPTER 6

The Self and Narcissism

The coparticipant inquiry into the nature of the personal self and the processes of self-fulfillment mirrors one of the central themes in post-Freudian psychoanalysis: the inquiry into narcissism. These two lines of inquiry share a similar concern with the psychology of the self. As Fairbairn (1952) tells us, people are fundamentally object-seeking, but they are also self-seeking, in search of their true selves. Beyond their shared concern with the self, however, self-actualization theorists and analysts who study narcissism take divergent paths, for they study very different selves. The study of narcissism is the inquiry into the interpersonal self, the "me" or reflected self. It is, in other words, the study of people's search for self-esteem—for interpersonal admiration, approval, and security. On the other hand, the study of self-fulfillment is the inquiry into the personal self, the "I" or self-generative and proactive self. It is the study of individuals' search for self-knowledge and self-expression.

As discussed earlier, the psychoanalytic theorist who has most fully explored this interpersonal dimension of the human psyche is the American interpersonal relations theorist Sullivan, whose study of the human psyche focused on the vicissitudes of the interpersonal self. The contemporary psychoanalytic study of narcissism, as exemplified in the work of Heinz Kohut and Otto Kernberg and numerous other post-Freudians, represents the contemporary analytic effort to study this same interpersonal dimension of the psyche in terms compatible with orthodox Freudian metapsychology.

Sullivan's focus on self-esteem, on man's search for interpersonal security led, however, to a truncated theory of self-actualizing man's search for personal fulfillment. This same bias also holds true for the post-Freudian theorists. Ironically, Kohut's (1971) concept of narcissism implicitly includes the theme of self-realization. Although self-actualization and narcissism represent opposite poles of self experience, Kohut's positing of a separate developmental line of narcissism, culminating in mature forms of narcissism, implies a dimension of selfness that is not interpersonal and not object-relational but is a self-seeking narcissism that is not self-centered. Kohut's complex concept of self-object relatedness and of a narcissistic line of psychological development refers to three different aspects of self-seeking: the search for interpersonal security, the seeking of relational intimacy, and the striving for self-fulfilling selfhood. Though Kohut's theorizing on narcissism may be seen to encompass an implicit self-actualization dynamic, he primarily focused on the clinical vicissitudes of the interpersonal, rather than the personal, self—that is, on the person as defined by his or her social surround.

Strivings for self-fulfillment are sometimes confused with pathologically narcissistic and pseudo-authentic forms of self-expression; thus, they may be seen as implying a disregard for the other. Quite the contrary is true. The actualization of one's capacities means that these capacities are lived in the relational as well as in the personal domains of experience. And though at times the pursuit of self-fulfillment may be lived in ways that incur social disapproval, it is neither hostile nor defensive; respect for otherness—for the individuality of others—is integral to its experience. The process of self-realization represents the antithesis of narcissistic self-absorption and self-alienation; it is born in respect and appreciation of one's own true potential and powers and implies respect for those of others.

The free expression of self-fulfilling strivings can be distinguished from the hurtful pseudo-authenticity that reveals itself in impulsive and compulsive defensive maneuvers. Patients often justify and rationalize acting out such defensive patterns of hostility and or interpersonal irresponsibility as freedom of self-expression in the service of "honesty," "truth," "authentic relatedness," or "telling it like it is." Such self-expression is, however, essentially a self-centered expression of narcissism, rather than a search for authentic speech or true selfness. In fact, defensiveness and hostility are the expression of a lack of selfness or self-actualization.

Narcissism thus may be defined as the perversion of self-realization. It is the self grown twisted and not rooted in itself. Self-estrangement and grandiose self-idealization (and its narcissistic twin, the idealization of others) are born when one's strivings for self-realization are stymied. Narcissistic pathology, such as a preoccupation with reflected self-esteem; strivings for superiority, power, and control; imperviousness to influence; and selfness defined by others represents the defensive perversion of self-actualizing strivings. It prevents the patient from being open to the unknown, from understanding himself or herself, and from loving and being close with others. Narcissism represents the rechanneling of the self-actualizing pursuit of personhood into the defensive pursuit of person-ahood. When efforts to live out one's true selfness and psychic capacities are stymied by anxiety, apprehension, and social pressures, they become defensively transformed into a narcissistic focus on a selfness that is rooted in the experience of the other, not in that of one's own being. Self-actualizing individuals are self- defining; however, narcissistic ones are simultaneously self-denying and self-deifying.

Both theoretically and clinically, narcissism has become a central concept in contemporary psychoanalytic inquiry, used increasingly by post-Freudians to define the fundamental human problems of *singularity*—the issues of self, individuality, and individuation—*relatedness*—questions of union, love, dependency, and community—*significance*—core concerns of self-esteem and self-love—and *limitation,* that is, questions of human imperfection, idealization, and finitude. This burgeoning interest in narcissism reflects a paradigmatic shift in psychoanalysis: the turn from drive to interpersonal to self theory and from an impersonal to interpersonal to personal model of analytic inquiry. This is evident in the growing awareness of the clinical centrality and therapeutic efficacy of coparticipatory forms of clinical inquiry.

The unifying thematic of narcissism, as a contemporary psychoanalytic concept is the self. The modern, post-Freudian study of narcissism and the self began with Freud's libidinal and economic theory of narcissism. Freud wrote his 1914 paper, "On Narcissism," as he was beginning to move from id theory and the topographical model to an ego psychology and structural model and intended it as a study of the processes of self-esteem and the formation of ideals as well as the processes of neurotic and psychotic introversion and megalomania (self-inflation). The paper was problematic for two reasons: First, Freud's U-tube hydraulic concept of narcissism in which a fixed amount of libidinal energy is reciprocally distributed between oneself and one's love interest, such that an increase in love for another means a decrease in self-love, and vice-versa has been contradicted in clinical practice. Freud's theory was logical, simple, even elegant, but empirically false. In real life, self-love and love for others are indivisible. As Fromm, one of the first critics of Freud's theory, points out, narcissism represents the opposite of both love of self and love of others. As Thompson notes, defensive clinical narcissism is self-hate, not self-love. In sum, defensive or clinical narcissism represents hateful, rather than loving, relatedness. Second, Freud's formulation failed to distinguish between quantity and quality, between bad self-love (defensive pride or pathological grandiosity and self-centeredness) and good self-love (healthy self-esteem), thus necessitating additional concepts in order to distinguish the various dimensions of narcissism.

After the paradigmatic shift from drive theory and impersonal concepts of therapy to an interpersonal (object relational) metapsychology and personal, coparticipatory, concepts of therapy, Freudian ego psychologists tried to correct for the deficiencies of Freud's libidinal theory of narcissism while remaining loyal to orthodox thought. They attempted to graft new concepts of the self onto a libidinal metapsychology not built to house them. Unfortunately, this has resulted in considerable conceptual (and terminological) confusion. While workable, the theory is conceptually cumbersome, as Kohut came to understand; therefore, he discarded the libidinal theory of narcissism and proposed a psychoanalytic self-psychology.

Adherents of nonorthodox psychoanalytic schools, such as the interpersonal and Horneyian schools, focused from the beginning on the study of the self and its social relations, making a significant contribution to the understanding of those phenomena we now call narcissistic. The theoretical and clinical contributions of these analysts antedated conceptions and therapeutic approaches mistakenly thought by many to have originated with contemporary Freudian theorists. These interpersonally oriented analysts traditionally placed problems of the self and narcissism at the center of their therapeutic inquiry (cf. Fromm 1964; Fiscalini and Grey 1993). The analytic study of patients' anxious interpersonal self (i.e., their "narcissistic" vulnerabilities and self-personifications) and defensive self-system functioning (what some call self-object relatedness) formed the center of their psychoanalytic work. The developmental history, analytic vicissitudes, and therapeutic transformation of patients' self-definition and sense of self is, for these heterodox analysts, central to therapeutic inquiry, as is the analytic play of such core defensive narcissistic processes as grandiosity, entitlement, and detachment.

Given that disorders of the self, rather than of the drives, have been the primary therapeutic variable in interpersonally oriented psychoanalytic treatment, these analysts historically have not focused on narcissism as a special clinical entity. Based on relational and self psychology, interpersonally oriented, particularly coparticipatory, psychoanalytic approaches to narcissistic phenomena have not found it necessary either to develop techniques special to working with narcissism—since these are already part of interpersonal coparticipatory psychoanalysis—nor to regard narcissism as qualitatively different from other forms of neurosis. Clinical observation suggests, in fact, that all patients have narcissistic problems in varying degrees. Narcissistic dynamics may be predominant or more severe in some patients—those who suffer from narcissistic personality disorders or borderline personalities. Nevertheless, such ways of relating characterize all patients to some extent. In other words, narcissism represents a type of problem rather than a type of person—a central dimension of psychopathology that cuts across the diagnostic spectrum.

The heterodox interpersonal relations analysts historically addressed the problems of clinical narcissism and disorders of the self in both their milder (neurotic) and more severe (psychotic) forms. Freud's division of the neuroses into the narcissistic and anaclitic and his view that the psychoses, the so-called the narcissistic neuroses, were unanalyzable because such patients are too self-absorbed to form a transference relationship, has proven clinically incorrect. This was amply demonstrated in the pioneering work of interpersonal psychoanalysts, such as Sullivan and Fromm-Reichmann, who successfully treated schizophrenia with a modified form of psychoanalysis; they proved that psychotic individuals are not detached and oblivious, but rather overstimulated interpersonally. Their analytic coparticipation is, in fact, dominated by transference relatedness and experience.

These interpersonal analysts used the participant-observation model of psychoanalytic inquiry—revolutionary at the time—and worked therapeutically with those narcissistic patients who, because of their difficulty in working within the strict limits of classical nonparticipant inquiry and their alleged inability to develop transference relationships, were judged by Freudian orthodoxy as psychoanalytically inaccessible—that is, impossible to analyze. Freud failed to see that these patients, though they did not manifest predominant Oedipal ties to the analyst, nevertheless showed strong and enduring transference attachments of a more primitive nature. In fact, as we now know, in cases of psychoses and character neuroses (including the so-called narcissistic personality), the clinical picture is dominated by such archaic transferences. The narcissism of these individuals represents the interpersonal warp of their disturbed early relationships with others. Withdrawal and narcissism, thus, are not inaccessible forms of self-engulfment or inverted libido, but primitive security dynamisms, ways of protecting a fragile and narcissistically injured interpersonal self. Though not responsive to classical impersonal inquiry, this self is therapeutically responsive to active and flexible interpersonal forms of coparticipant clinical inquiry.

Similarly, Freudians' division of patients into those with so-called developmentally arrested (pre-oedipal) self-disorders and those with psychically conflicted (oedipal) drive problems is a spurious and unnecessary dichotomy that springs from the theoretical desire to graft a psychology of the self onto a libidinal metapsychology. Interpersonally oriented psychoanalytic approaches do not require such an empirically inaccurate division. In fact, early narcissistic experiences and anxieties inevitably result in intertwined concerns with both arrested (or warped) growth and intrapsychic conflict, that is, in persisting residuals of unmet developmental narcissistic needs (e.g., mirroring or idealizing needs) and in learned patterns of defensive narcissism.

The formulations of Kohut's psychology of the self and those of his followers represent the most focused effort to establish such a theory compatible with Freudian orthodoxy. Despite initial efforts to conceptualize the self and narcissistic processes in libidinal terms, Kohut increasingly found this unsatisfactory and eventually abandoned attempts to define the self and its many dimensions in terms of the concept of narcissism. Instead, like the cultural-interpersonal analysts before him, he developed an explicit theory of the interpersonal self in which his findings were interpreted in terms of the concept of self-object relatedness. Thus, for example, the so-called narcissistic personality disorders became known as disorders of self-object relations. In fact, Kohut eventually stood traditional nosology on its head by defining all psychopathology, even the Oedipus complex, in terms of self-psychology. What had started out as a libido theory of narcissism thus became a study of the self and its discontents.

Kohut's new nosology was foreshadowed in Horney's work. In her final schema of neurotic character structure (Horney 1950), all neurosis is seen as inherently narcissistic, and neurotics are described as having developed self-contradictory defensive character trends. This leads to inner conflicts and a comprehensive neurotic solution by compensatory processes of defensive self-idealization involving an *idealized image*, a *search for glory*—that is, an attempt to actualize the defensive *idealized self*—and contempt toward the *real self*. This psychodynamic schema, which bears a formal similarity to Kernberg's theory of borderline/narcissistic dynamics, outlines various neurotic forms of the search for glory, including a specific character type that is similar to Kohut's narcissistic personality disorder. Realizing the clinical centrality of defensive self-idealization, Horney classified all neurosis as fundamentally narcissistic—as signs of self-alienation and compensatory grandiosity. Like Erich Fromm, Horney emphasized that narcissism was essentially self-alienation, a divorce of the person from his or her creative capacities and sense of being. Horney and Fromm, like Winnicott, spoke of a "real" or "true" self whose development is stunted in the pathological narcissistic process. Horney's work, however, has not received the attention it deserves, and its influence has been relatively limited, largely because she and her followers worked outside of the psychoanalytic mainstream and now form a relatively small and less influential psychoanalytic tributary. Kohut's work, on the other hand, lies largely within mainstream psychoanalysis (though it has required complex theoretical gyrations to maintain its metapsychological ties to orthodoxy), and thus it has had a broader, albeit not necessarily more original, impact on the wider psychoanalytic community.

Kohut's central contribution to psychoanalysis is that he provided Freudian orthodoxy with the theoretical means for working analytically with patients previously thought not susceptible to analysis. Traditionally, Freudian analysts considered only patients who could form a stable Oedipal transference neurosis as capable of analytic treatment. Not infrequently, narcissistic patients with marked self-esteem vulnerability were misidentified as Oedipal patients with unresolvable narcissistic resistances. However, Kohut's formulation of the narcissistic "mirroring" and "idealizing" transferences expanded Freudian metapsychology to include the interpersonal self and thereby legitimized neoclassical analytic work with problems of narcissism and the self. Kohut interpersonalized Freudian metapsychology, but not its clinical methodology. His achievement was not a radical restructuring of psychoanalytic technique, but rather a broadening of its interpretive range.

Kohut's formulation of the self-object transferences called orthodox attention to the interpsychic dimension of all transferences. Self-object relatedness, as conceptualized by Kohut, refers to the psychic dimension Sullivan called the need for interpersonal security. I refer to it as the domain of the interpersonal self—the innate human need for acceptance and interpersonal approval, or esteem. Kohut's self-object is essentially Sullivan's reflecting appraiser—the interpersonal arbiter of the representational, or reflected, self. Thus, self-object transferences represent not a special kind of transference characteristic of only certain patients, but rather a central, interpsychic, dimension of all transference structures. Self-object needs differ, however, in their specific content and nature, ranging from archaic security requirements of a more primitive narcissistic nature to more mature forms of the need for interpersonal approval and security. In other words, the interpersonal self dimension of transference experience exists on a developmental continuum.

Self-object transferences, as defined by Kohut drew the attention of orthodox theorists to the frequently archaic nature of parataxic relatedness. These primitive self-object transferences and countertransferences represent the repetition of early narcissistic aspects of the "not-me" selfpersonification. They arise from traumatic interpersonal experiences of early needs for relational intimacy, personal fulfillment, or physical satisfaction. In the analytic situation, these unmet narcissistic needs are symbolized and enacted in transferential bids for analytic approval in primitive mirroring and idealizing terms. These narcissistic transference paradigms do not differ in outline, but only in dynamic and developmental detail, from other more mature ones, such as the classical Oedipal transference. Like any other transference paradigm, they reflect arrested and dissociated personal and interpersonal experience that clinically presents itself as an integral of unconscious need, anxiety, and a defensive (self-protective) process.

Interpersonally or culturally oriented psychoanalysts focus on the self and its interpersonal relations and have not found it necessary to discover the narcissistic transferences for the analytic study of problems of the self. Traditionally considering all neuroses disorders of the self, they do not need to distinguish two discontinuous sets of clinical transferences: oedipal for drive disorders and narcissistic for disorders of the self. Repudiating narrow orthodox definitions of the psychoanalytic situation, these heterodox psychoanalysts have considered all neuroses as treatable with psychoanalysis.

Though Kohut's work on the self and narcissism was preceded by that of the interpersonal theorists, his influence on contemporary Freudian conceptions of the psychopathology of the self has been profound. Though the interpersonal self, or self-object relatedness, forms an integral aspect of all transference configurations, it is clinically most apparent in its more primitive forms, and thus this aspect of the transference dominates the clinical picture Kohut describes. In these cases, patients' need for approval is so great and experienced in such developmentally archaic ways that it both rules and defines his or her analytic coparticipation. Kohut's contribution to psychoanalytic thought and practice consists in his detailed study of these primitive transferences, which characterize all patients (and analysts) to some extent. In his studies of narcissism, Kohut broadened our analytic understanding of how early problems in reflected interpersonal appraisals can cripple subsequent living among others. As a clinician, Kohut was keenly sensitive to the extreme vulnerability of self-esteem—the marked sensitivity to real or imagined disapproval—of his "narcissistic" patients, and he realized that hearing their characterological narcissism empathically was crucial to the analysis of their repressed and injured interpersonal selves.

CHAPTER 7

Clinical Narcissism
Psychopathology of the Self

Narcissism is an ancient form of human suffering. The psychological and spiritual perils of self-absorption and human arrogance are told in the sacred writings of our most ancient religions. Thus the understanding of the moral, social, and personal dangers of solipsistic self-rapture and self-blinding vanity reaches back in time, farther even than that of the Greek mythology that names this all-too-common affliction.

Narcissistic relatedness, symbolized dramatically by the self-enraptured plight of mythic Narcissus, is the plight of the unloved self. The pathology of narcissism is the psychopathology of the self, in particular that dimension of the self that Sullivan refers to as the sum of reflected appraisals and that Kohut calls self-object relatedness and that I define as the domain of the interpersonal self. These various perspectives point to the dimension of personality that defines the need for interpersonal security—the human need for social approval or communal acceptance. Narcissism and self-inflation, in other words, represent a defensive substitute for healthy self-esteem.

Clinical narcissism, the defensive development of pathological grandiosity and self-centeredness, also figures in the psychopathology of the personal self; it is inimical to the free development and availability of the personal self. In fact, it could be said that clinical narcissism represents the pathological truncating of the personal self and traumatizing of the interpersonal self.

Moving from the time of ancient civilizations to the relatively recent history of the psychoanalytic exploration of the human psyche, we encounter a rise in recent years in the diagnosis of pathological or clinical narcissism, of what, in Kohut's diagnostic terms, are called the disorders of the self.

This phenomenon prompts two questions: First, is there an actual increase in this form of problematic living? Is this a phenomenon of new pathology or one of new nosology, of a change in our perception of our patients? Does this increase reveal a new understanding of an old problem, rather than the birth of a new problem? Second, does the recent diagnostic frequency of the narcissistic personality disorder, whether reflective of new pathology or of new nosology, represent a class of human psychic distress and disturbance that is uniquely self-disordered, qualitatively different from classical neuroses and personality disorders? Many analytic theorists, particularly Freudians, hold that narcissistic pathology is a unique, developmentally arrested disorder of the self, unlike Oedipal neuroses, which are psychosexually fixated drive disorders.

Many cultural critics, such as Christopher Lasch (1979), argue that narcissism is on the rise in our contemporary Western culture, reflecting the pathological deterioration of our society. Clearly, pathological trends in our modern society are in many ways psychologically conducive to the growth of narcissistic disorders. Nevertheless, inquiry into our diagnostics of as much as fifty years ago suggests that narcissism was as frequent then as it is now. Then, however, it was labeled differently. Today's narcissistic personality, so commonly found following the introduction of Kohut's ideas, was formerly subsumed under the categories of hysteric, schizoid, obsessive, depressive, or paranoid. Thus, Lasch's (1979) narcissistic personality of today is more or less identical to Horney's (1937) neurotic personality of yesterday: self-centered, competitive, constantly striving for power and prestige and perfection, insatiable, hostile, anxious, and overly sensitive to rejection. Consider Horney's words, written over sixty-five years ago:

> Narcissistic trends are frequent in our culture. More often than not people are incapable of true friendship and love; they are egocentric . . . they feel insecure and tend to overrate their personal significance; they lack judgment of their own value because they have relegated it to others. (1939, p. 98)

Looking even farther back in time, we find narcissistic or borderline patients among Freud's hysterics. Pathological trends in our contemporary culture, such as our excessive materialism, focus on instant gratification, preoccupation with prestige and status, and competitiveness, clearly contribute to the development of narcissistic processes, perhaps even to the point where we might be justified in calling the U.S. a narcissistic nation. However, I think that the increased frequency of this diagnosis is due primarily to a shift in our nosological paradigm from drive psychology to a psychoanalytic emphasis on the self and its social relations. That is, there has been a change in our perceptions of our patients rather than in our patients themselves.

Moreover, the patients with disorders of the self now labeled narcissistic are not fundamentally different in kind from those with oedipal neuroses, that is, with disorders of the drives. Contemporary Freudian theorists's insistence on such a diagnostic bifurcation reflects their complicated attempt to somehow preserve the libido theory while also acknowledging the insights of interpersonal and object relational theories. However, this dichotomy does not hold up in clinical practice. Rather, as Sullivan posited and Kohut agreed, all personality disorders are disorders of the self, regardless of the level of disturbance and the nature of the predominant character structure. In this sense, narcissism may be said to be a universal process, an essential aspect of all psychic disturbance. Clinical observation suggests that all patients exhibit a narcissistic core. Though narcissistic dynamics may be predominant or more severe in some patients—those whom we diagnose as having narcissistic personality disorders or borderline personalities—such ways of relating characterize all patients to some degree.

Narcissism comprises a complex set of clinical features that form what may be called a *core narcissistic constellation,* characterized by the following defensive dynamics: (1) self-centeredness and lack of empathy for others; (2) grandiosity; (3) cyclic contempt and idealization of both oneself and others; (4) thick-headedness or psychological inaccessibility and imperviousness; (5) thin-skinnedness or abnormal vulnerability of self-esteem; (6) attitudes of entitlement to special rights or privileges; (7) other-directedness or the ceaseless search for the approval, admiration, attention, and acceptance from others; and (8) power orientation—striving for control and coerciveness.

This constellation of narcissistic defenses underlies all neurotic functioning and all psychopathology. This *core narcissistic constellation* bears a striking similarity to many of the central clinical features of Guntrip's (1969) schizoid, Sullivan's (1956) hysteric, Salzman's (1980) obsessional, and Bonime's (1982a,b) depressive and paranoid categories.

People are narcissistic in three ways: first, we all have problems with self-esteem; second, this problem with self-esteem inevitably involves deficits in so-called normal narcissism. All of us carry archaic needs for validation of self-esteem that are based on grandiosity and express themselves in what Kohut calls "mirroring" and "idealizing" needs. Third, we all develop pathological narcissistic defenses or security operations. Thus, all patients and analysts have problems with narcissism. Some people, however, are so predominantly characterized by narcissistic defensive traits that we refer to them as narcissistic personalities. In other words, all patients have narcissistic problems, and some more so than others. Thus, we can speak of the coparticipant analysis of narcissistic processes in every patient's treatment and of the coparticipant analytic treatment of the narcissist—the person or personality who presents a predominance of narcissistic dynamics and traits.

THE CORE NARCISSISTIC CONSTELLATION

Self-Centeredness. Let us briefly review these dynamics. First, let us consider the single most defining feature of the core narcissistic constellation: self-centeredness. Comprising conscious and unconscious interpersonal attitudes and behaviors such as exhibitionism, egoism, selfishness, vanity, and imperviousness to influence, self-centeredness includes a broad spectrum of self-referential processes. The more narcissistic one is, the more others are experienced as undifferentiated extensions of oneself.

The narcissistic individual is unable or unwilling to open himself or herself to seeing others as persons in their own right and to empathically relate to their needs or desires. As Fromm (1973) observes, narcissism "is a state of experience in which only the person himself, *his* body, *his* needs, *his* feelings, *his* thoughts, *his* property . . . are experienced as fully real, while everybody and everything that does not form part of the person or is not an object of his needs is . . . *affectively* without weight and color" (p. 201). For the narcissist, others exist only as insubstantial shadows or reflections of one's narcissistic self. Sullivan (1956), too, sees the narcissistic individual as living in a "lotus-land sort of existence" (p. 212) in which others "have no real importance . . . except as an audience," i.e., as idealized or mirroring self-objects.

Self-centeredness represents, of course, the absence of a centered self. Narcissistic individuals are focused on maintaining or bolstering an insecure interpersonal self—preoccupied with securing a sense of self-esteem, usually in grandiose terms. Individuals preoccupied with obtaining "narcissistic supplies"—admiration, approval, attention, etc.—are often very sensitive to, and disparaging of, similar traits in others. Marriages are often characterized by patterns of coparticipation in which each mate is very sensitive to the partner's self-centeredness, while remaining blind to his or her own.

Sullivan (1940) describes a "self-absorbed" personality syndrome in which there is "a cosmic centering in the person" and experience is largely bifurcated in terms of the primitive early childhood pattern of good-mother and bad, or evil, mother (p. 78). Sullivan described these persons as particularly apt to become "disappointed, wounded, or misunderstood" in their relations with those whom they cannot idealize. He sardonically added that "one cannot but marvel at the failure of learning which has left their capacity for fantastic, self-centered illusion so utterly unaffected by a life-long series of educative events"(p. 80). Fromm (1947) contrasts the self-infatuation of narcissism with the ability to truly love oneself and others. For Fromm, love is a relationship of one-ness with others that is based upon a recognition of their and one's own individuality and integrity.

Self-centered individuals protect against feelings of dependency and their needs for tenderness and help by efforts at superhuman self-control or control over others. Imperviousness, detachment, and dissociation of the need for tenderness (Pearce and Newton 1963) may be seen as coercive power operations designed to protect against unconscious feelings and fears of helplessness, inadequacy, or insignificance. Such narcissistic efforts at control inhibit one's openness, ability to engage in give-and-take and to "surrender" (Horney 1937) to oneself or another; they markedly impair one's interpersonal relations and experience of the world.

For the narcissist, admitting that he or she needs others or is open to their influence carries the psychic risk of a humiliating or frightening acknowledgment of human vulnerability and emotional interdependency.

Grandiosity. Defensive grandiosity, the pathological search for perfection, power, or superiority may exist on varying levels of awareness. It may be overtly evidenced in conscious feelings of superiority and special entitlement. Often, however, the more troublesome aspects of grandiosity are lived out unconsciously. Covert grandiose beliefs or tendencies may be hidden by overt dependency, timidity, or passivity.

Grandiosity ranges in the level of distortion or self-inflation from the megalomaniacal fantasies of the psychotic through the grandiose illusions of the narcissist to the narcissistic conceits seen in everyone (what may be called the grandiosity of everyday life). The grandiose individual feels acceptable only when admired or approved by others; criticism, of course, is anathema.

The grandiose individual engages in a ceaseless "search for glory" and for narcissistic affirmation of his or her grandiose self. Narcissistic individuals need to constantly buttress their grandiose selves by repeatedly proving their omnipotence, omniscience, superiority, or perfection. Thus, in various interpersonal contexts defensive narcissistic needs to exploit, dominate, humiliate, or in other ways prevail over all others and all limits become psychologically mandatory. Such power operations become dynamically ever more necessary, with major efforts directed to coercing others into narcissistically needed interactions.

The grandiose narcissist always lives on the brink of anxiety and narcissistic mortification. The more grandiose a person, the more vulnerable to criticism and disapproval he or she is. Grandiose individuals, driven by their narcissistic anxieties and vulnerabilities, seek increasing refuge in their grandiose illusions. A narcissistic spiral eventuates: increasing self-alienation and self-contempt leading to increased narcissistic grandiosity leading to greater, and more vulnerable, narcissistic demands for admiration, leading to increasingly more vulnerable self-esteem, and so on.

Learned by example (identification) and by trial and error, grandiose self-inflation is a precarious defense in that reality often points to its unrealistic foundations, thus exposing the person to a humiliating brush with his or her real limitations. Like all defenses, grandiosity involves the denial of reality, which at times extends to a refusal to observe the laws of cause and effect, thus interfering with safety or success in living. Grandiose self-inflation may prompt vain or even self-destructive attempts to live up to one's defensively inflated expectations.

Though grandiosity is designed to compensate for self-contempt derived from early interpersonal experience, it actually serves to weaken one's self-regard. When the defensively grandiose self becomes the measure of approval (the standard for self-esteem), then the actual self becomes an object of contempt. Thus, the grandiose narcissist's self-esteem is always a fragile matter, and shame and hints of nightmarish uncanny emotion are perceived as threats. In its demands the grandiose interpersonal self, the narcissistic means of security, becomes itself a potential source of shame and self-loathing. For the narcissist, shortcomings, whether clearly perceived or only vaguely felt, are inevitably experienced as humiliating. Even success may feel like failure because it doesn't measure up to the narcissist's irrational expectations. Thus the slightest criticism, neglect, or absence of special recognition becomes a shameful and humiliating experience, a narcissistic insult or blow to one's self-esteem. The relation of grandiose self-inflation to a void in self-esteem is obvious, and the brittleness of this defense is readily apparent to clinical scrutiny.

Direct confrontation of one's self-inflation can spark latent anxiety and result in reactive hostility, often marked by the defensive use of narcissistic rage, a sure sign of wounded grandiosity. The anger provoked by threats to one's narcissistic equilibrium cannot remove the personal source of narcissistic anxiety or shame, but it erases, at least temporarily, the experience of it and obscures the damage to one's self-esteem. Almost everyone prefers anger to the experience of anxiety—being angry to feeling weak, subhuman, or loathsomely inferior. These are the feelings of the self-inflated narcissist when his or her grandiose ambitions are punctured. The fear of such "narcissistic collapse" often drives narcissists to redouble their grandiose strivings, reinforcing their imperviousness and increasing their controlling-ness in their effort to bend reality to conform to their grandiose self-images.

Idealization. Idealization of others often coexists with narcissistic self-aggrandizement. The narcissistic pursuit of power and perfection is then found in union (symbiotic identification) with the admired other. This defensive dynamic differs from children's developmentally appropriate "naive" idealization of their parents. Early harsh, developmentally misattuned, interpersonal experience inevitably results in both pathological defensive idealizations of others and repressed and unrequited childlike adoration and admiration of the parent (persisting "idealized" infantile parent imagos), which are lived out in the "idealizing" component of transferential relations.

The defensive search for idealized others originates in an unconscious sense of weakness and vulnerability. Elicited by the fear of self-initiative, independent action, or individual expression of wish or feeling, it is the desire to find safety in identification or merger with the defensively idealized parent.

Narcissistic individuals are prone to oscillate between devaluation and idealization of themselves and others. This unhappy dynamic results from the ready tendency of narcissistic individuals to focus on others' and their own failure to live up to impossible grandiose standards. These individuals are chronically "disappointed" with both others and themselves. Both self-inflation and idealization of others are fragile processes. This might not seem so to the coparticipant analyst who must contend with another feature of narcissistic functioning: imperviousness to influence.

The narcissistic person is both thick-headed and thin-skinned. Narcissistic individuals almost automatically refuse or refute the input from others. Narcissists are deeply fearful of open contact with others, for this portends the disorganization of their narcissistic personas. While narcissistic patients may be difficult to reach, they are at the same time thin-skinned, overly vulnerable to insult or disapproval.

Narcissistic individuals may form mutual admiration societies or symbiotic dependencies, which may last a lifetime, often insidiously developing into "hostile integrations" or sadomasochistic relationships. The more timid narcissists who repress their own arrogance tend to admire and to be attracted to the seeming self-assurance, and sense of certainty of overtly arrogant and exhibitionistic narcissists who often exude a kind of narcissistic charisma. In their symbiotic union narcissists are trying to transcend the terrifying anxiety they associate with unique individuality. This narcissistic flight into the illusory perfection of sadomasochistic and symbiotic relatedness represents an escape from the freedom and responsibility of realizing one's true, separate selfness, a turning away from the responsibilities and possibilities of the personal self.

Entitlement and Demandingness. Overtly or covertly, narcissistic individuals tend to demand and often extract privileges, assistance, or special treatment from others. The loud, spoiled demands of the overtly arrogant narcissist simply represent the most obvious form of entitlement. Much more frequently, such attitudes are hidden. This attitude of irrational entitlement represents the narcissistic trait that people dislike most and have most difficulty with. Such a demanding attitude invariably places great strains on interpersonal integrations and becomes a frequent reason for social (or therapeutic) rejection of the narcissist. Such narcissistic people are poorly tolerated unless they possess some special gift or quality. Those with unusual beauty, wealth, fame, power, or personal charisma are likely to be idealized and treated with special care. However, the arrogation of special privilege, as manifested in unreasonable demands for service, combined with personal conceit and arrogance will after a while exhaust the patience and empathy of even the most stoic persons. Herein, of course, lies great potential for provocation of disjunctive countertransference experience in the psychoanalytic situation.

Narcissists' grandiose presumption of special privilege or prerogative, together with their repudiation of personal responsibility, social reciprocity, and interpersonal empathy inevitably vexes and alienates other people. Their demanding attitude may lead to the disintegration of interpersonal situations that might otherwise have proved satisfactory to all coparticipants.

The refusal, or inability, to meet the narcissist's inordinate and inappropriate demands almost always provokes feelings of angry disappointment and projective accusations of insensitivity or hostility. Insatiable demands for unconditional love, however masked, often characterize the narcissist's relations with others. They represent the defensive demand for relatedness without reciprocity or responsibility—relationship as a one-way street.

The defensive other side of narcissists' interpersonal coerciveness and demanding stance is their rejection of any requests or expectations others make of them. Others' requests often are projectively experienced by narcissists as coercive attempts for control. Insisting on having what they want when they want it and in the way that they want it, narcissists resent any abridgment of what they consider their freedom to do as they wish.

Other-directedness and Self-alienation. Driven by their vulnerable self-esteem, compensatory grandiosity, and defensive idealization of others, narcissistic individuals alienate themselves not only from others but also from themselves—from their own deeper being and psychic center. Narcissistic individuals are focused on their interpersonal selves, i.e., on the social pursuit of interpersonal security, to the point of eclipsing their personal selves or unique individuality.

Patients' narcissistic dependency on others is seen in their other-directedness—in their constant search for validation and mirroring approval from others. For the narcissist, self-esteem is determined by the willingness of others to reflect positive appraisals of oneself. One's interpersonal self is thus a reflection of other reflected selves.

Other-directedness implies self-alienation. All experience is colored, and hence altered, by the need for approval from others. The narcissist's self-centeredness, in other words, is an uncentered selfness, a self alienated from itself. May (1953) considers such narcissistic other-directedness as typical of many people in modern American (or Western) culture and refers to such narcissistically oriented individuals as the hollow people. Since for these individuals self-esteem is based on outside approval, it tends to vary with changes in the social environment. The narcissistic person thus is much like a rudderless ship, at the mercy of external circumstances, pushed and pulled by the shifts and swirls of interpersonal wind and tide.

Whether they strive for interpersonal affirmation in arrogant or in appeasing ways, narcissistic individuals are almost wholly dependent on others for reflected approval and definition. For the narcissist, self-esteem and self-integrity are externally regulated, dependent on the interpersonal mirroring of idealized others.

Narcissists seek others' approval because they lack autonomous standards for self-evaluation and self-validation. They are alienated from their direct experience of their desires, intuitions, and feelings. In a sense, the narcissist may be said to be overly interpersonalized or overly adapted. May (1953) refers to this aspect of narcissism when he speaks of the contemporary "radar" type of person who "lives as though he were directed by a radar set . . . perpetually telling him what others expect" and "gets his motive and directions from others . . . able to respond but not to choose; he has no effective center of motivation of his own" (p. 19). The search for specialness, the compulsive and relatively indiscriminate narcissistic drive for praise and approval, is always at the expense of one's own true potential. The narcissist's personal development is invariably truncated. As May (1953) reminds us, narcissism inevitably involves a "betrayal of one's self" (p. 235). Early experiences of anxiety and social pressure defensively shunt or transform the effort to live out one's psychic capacities into a narcissistic focus on a selfness that is rooted in the other, not in oneself.

When any of the dynamics sketched here show signs of failing and not working their magic, the narcissistic individual will often generate irritation, anger, or rage, along with an intensification of his or her narcissistic strategies to achieve the defensive safety of feelings of perfection, specialness, symbiotic "love," and exemption from personal consequence and responsibility. Though these dynamics may be predominant or more severe in some patients—those we diagnose as having narcissistic personality disorders or borderline conditions—such ways of relating characterize all patients to some degree.

THOUGHTS ON DIAGNOSIS

Individuals are usually consistent in their behavior and experience. But character has complexity as well as consistency. We are all much more complex than generally assumed—including in our narcissistic facets—and our relatedness to others and to ourselves, narcissistic and otherwise, varies with its coparticipant context, with the situation, time, and person(s) to whom we are relating.

Doubtless all patients and analysts are complex and individual integrals of various personality trends. The various dynamics characterizing the various diagnostic categories—e.g., obsessionalism, hysteria, paranoia, narcissism, etc.—represent processes, capacities, or ways of being and relating that are universal, and they typify us all in some aspect of our living, even if only to a very minor extent. Each of us represents a unique category, a certain individual pattern, of all these dynamics though we may be predominantly this or that sort of personality. We are all mixed neurotics, even those of us who appear more nearly to approximate a pure type. Diagnostic categories are neither truly discrete nor even real entities; they are simply names given to certain identified clinical features.

Even though we may simply be human like all other people, as Sullivan (1940) reminds us, we are also very individual in our humanity. Even in our narcissism—the very antithesis of unique individuality—we are unique. And just as hysterics, obsessionals, depressives, etc. represent heterogeneous groups, so do narcissists. A patient may be more narcissistic than otherwise, but his or her narcissism is always uniquely patterned. There is great heterogeneity among narcissists in the nature, pattern, dynamics, and pathogenetic paths of their narcissism. Patients vary in their narcissism depending on the severity, frequency, extent, and individual patterning of their narcissistic concerns and problems.

With the narcissist, as with any patient, therapy requires that the individual be understood in his or her true singularity, in his or her specific and unique psychic needs and experiences.

THE DEVELOPMENTAL EMERGENCE OF NARCISSISM

How does one become narcissistic? Is there a specific developmental path for narcissism, a particular set of experiences that predispose an individual toward narcissistic ways of being and relating? Notwithstanding the procrustean implications of such typology, four etiological patterns of narcissism may be identified. We may call them: the *shamed child*, the *spoiled child*, the *special child*, and the *spurned child*.

This typology is a heuristic, offered as a way of examining significant aspects of the development of narcissistic processes and problems. These four etiological patterns outlined here are highly abstract, schematic representations of what, in actuality, are complex series of interpersonal interactions and personal experiences that are lived out in a multitude of individual ways. The shamed, spoiled, special, and spurned child each refer to countless interpersonal interactions that involve complexly intertwined needs and desires of both parent and child. This etiological schema represents an introductory outline of those interpersonal experiences that I think are most central in the formation of narcissistic pathology—an abstract, as it were, of some important developmental vicissitudes of the interpersonal self.

The child who develops a solid, realistic, and personally grounded sense of security or self-esteem—so-called healthy narcissism—requires a social environment in which both unconditional and conditional love and approval are provided appropriately by the parenting figures. Very young children require mirroring or loving approval, which from an adult perspective may seem extravagant or extreme, for activities or being-states that later on in the child's development will be responded to in a more modulated way. For example, parents may adore or admire their child for some seemingly ordinary action or interaction—a smile, a spoken word, enthusiasm, an expression of some desire—or cherish him or her for simply being alive.

This early unconditional cherishing of the infant and young child in conjunction with the parent's enjoyment and acceptance of the child's reciprocal admiration constitutes the wordless foundation of all later self-esteem. It forms the nonverbal core of the interpersonal self. It becomes internalized as the child's own strong and primal sense of confirmed personal worthiness. Its absence, what Balint (1968) might call the "basic fault" and what we observe in patients as a vague, elusive sense of "wrongness" or "badness"—of being somehow defective or no good, is rooted in early deficits of mirroring in this preverbal time. This difficulty is often refractory to verbal intervention and needs to be worked though analytically in what I have called the "living through process" (Fiscalini 1988).

As the child matures in cognitive and emotional capacity, parents' reflective approval becomes conditional, both more tempered and more selectively offered and received. There is, in other words, a gradual limiting or disillusioning of the previously "unbounded self"—the egocentric and naively grandiose child—and, reciprocally, of the primitively idealized parent. When the socialization or child-rearing process, including the setting of limits, is consistently applied and commensurate with the maturational capacities of the child and his or her personal abilities and limitations, it will result in a realistic and robust self-esteem, increased awareness of and empathy for others, and autonomous standards for self-evaluation.

The Shamed Child. When children experience chronic disapproval of significant aspects of their developmentally appropriate attachment (loving), dependency, or individuating needs because of parental anxiety, envy, jealousy, or hatred, they will grow up feeling shameful and fearful and inadequate in these areas of their psyche. Even their very need to receive approval or mirroring and to approve of or idealize the parent may become shamefully unacceptable. These shameful, anxious aspects of the psyche are dissociated and become part of the "not-me" aspect of the personality. The shamed child's relationship with his or her parent is characterized by unempathic harshness and an unempathic and excessive setting of limits and expectations. The parent anxiously or angrily demands that the child be more mature or grown-up than he or she can be. Too much is expected of the child.

The shamed child develops grandiose or unrealistic self-expectations that somehow he or she *should* or *could* or even *must* be more or better or different than his or her rejected actuality. The child feels "bad" or "wrong"—in some way difficult to verbalize not good enough. If the injury to the child's interpersonal self (self-esteem) is broad and deep, the child may later spend most of his or her adult life searching for security rather than for satisfying, fulfilling, or loving experiences. What characteristics of the child incur parental disapproval varies: any human capacity or need may be subject to interpersonal rejection and repudiation.

The persisting unmirrored needs of the child are often found in symptomatic activity—e.g., compulsive or addictive behaviors, defensive searches for glory—or in an aching, hard to voice, sense of unworthiness. The shamed child's experience is marked by a residual longing for approval of the rejected aspects of his or her psyche. This can be as specific, for example, as an unconscious longing to have one's athleticism or artistic talent appreciated. Or it can be more general, as in unconscious longings for affirmation of one's feelings of accomplishment, experiences of pleasure, or dependent wishes to be "babied" and tenderly cared for. Most primitively, there may be persisting needs for approval of one's self, one's very aliveness—to simply "be" and to be cherished for that "being."

The substitutive security operations, or character defenses, of the shamed child are those modeled or permitted in the home, whether masochism, depression, obsessionalism, sadism, or others.

The etiological pattern of the shamed child, when it is the predominant one in the developmental mix, fits the clinical picture of the shy or timid narcissist. These are the patients who might be diagnosed by some analysts (certainly by Kohutians) as narcissists, but would be diagnosed by others as obsessive, depressive, schizoid, or paranoid. The defensive narcissism tends to be covert, hidden behind other character defenses, as are the persisting aspects of the personality that remain unmirrored and unloved.

The Spoiled Child. Not infrequently, parents will indulge their children and fail to modify their approval to their developing maturity. This "protracted illusionment" of the child's egocentricity and naive grandiosity expresses itself in two subpatterns: *the uncivilized child* and *the infantilized child*.

Parents of the uncivilized child are overly lenient and fail to set appropriate limits or expectations for the child. Often the child is treated as though he or she were a young prince or princess. The parents overpraise their child and fail to establish conditions for approval that are tied to the child's real abilities. There is much "untamed" grandiosity and idealization in this situation. This leads to demanding and self-centered despotic behaviors and feelings of anger and rage when the person is treated as ordinary. Feelings of inadequacy or anxious inferiority emerge when the individual runs into realistic difficulty, reversal, or failure, since grandiose self-expectations have been built up by the parents' inflated appraisals. This child is not properly prepared for real life.

Indulgence, of course, always implies deprivation. When a child is excessively admired, some real aspects of the child are neglected. These unmirrored or disapproved needs, parts of the actual self, become repressed and part of the "not-me" and persist unconsciously as childhood narcissism into adulthood. Spoiling or indulgent over-evaluation of the child implies a parental inability to tolerate the child's needs to be independently effective. It also implies a rejection of both the child's real limitations and his or her developmental needs for limits and realistic appraisals.

The pattern of the infantilized child is substantially similar in its narcissistic dynamics to that of the uncivilized child, but it has a different, less aggressive or hostile, emotional tone and manifests in a different clinical picture later on. Narcissism is created here by parental overprotection and overly "sensitive" treatment of the "fragile" and precious child. This often coexists with excessive parental control and domination (as, for example, in the "Big Daddy" or "Big Momma" syndromes), which is denied and often rationalized as caring or loving concern. As an adult, the infantilized child is dependent, timid, and fearful of individuation and separation. This child is cherished and generally approved of but not released to independent living.

The spoiled child manifests both overt and covert defensive narcissism. In contrast to the uncivilized child, the overly sensitive infantilized child's defensive narcissism is more masked, less angrily demanded, and more idealizing. Clinically, the intertwined subtypes of the spoiled child are always mixed with aspects of the shamed child. Depending on the particular etiological patterning and its narcissistic severity, the patient may be diagnosed as a narcissist or as suffering from one of the other neuroses— often as an hysteric, depressive, dependent, or inadequate personality when the spoiled picture is predominant; all this depends, of course, on the nature of the character defenses adopted. In the case of very severe problems with being civilized, particularly when linked with severe shaming, symptoms may include acting-out or psychopathic features. In all of these clinical pictures, there is overt defensive, i.e., pathological, narcissism, which has been learned in the faulty interactive patterns of the spoiled child. This defensive characterological narcissism masks but should not to be mistaken for the repressed and unmirrored loving, expanding, and individuating needs of the young child.

The Special Child. This pattern of parent-child interaction combines aspects of the shamed child with a variant of the spoiled child. This etiological dynamic typifies patients who are most commonly diagnosed as having narcissistic personalities, including many of Kernberg's narcissists, Kohut's noisy or demanding narcissists, and Kohut's (1979) case of Mr. Z.

As with the shamed child, the parents of the special child are often rejecting: too busy, moralistic, competitive, envious, angry, anxious, perfectionist, or otherwise self-preoccupied to relate and respond to their child's developmentally appropriate needs for attention, admiration, acceptance, and affirmation in significant dimensions of their living. But unlike the shamed child, the special child is also highly prized, spoiled in self-centered ways, and used narcissistically, by the parent. In this situation, the parent, because of his or her narcissism, prizes the child for ways of being that are construed by the parent as bringing glory or reflected self-esteem to him or her. Thus, special or superior qualities, achievements, abilities, or talents are "over-mirrored" and become the selective basis for the child's self-esteem. These special qualities may be real or illusory; in either case, a *false self* is rewarded and simultaneously the *real self* is disparaged and remains largely unloved and unadmired.

The developmental experience of the special child leads to compulsive strivings for success, feelings of specialness, demands for praise and special treatment, and manifest arrogance. And, inevitably, secret fears of inferiority and inadequacy follow.

The mismirrored special child ends up feeling special, yet not worthwhile. The child gets what he or she doesn't need and doesn't get what he or she needs. Unconscious longings for mirroring from an ideal, caring parent coexist with manifest narcissistic pathology stemming from parental misapproval. Loved only for his or her special features and not for his or her real being, the special child grows into the archetypal narcissist—only secure interpersonally when experiencing himself or herself as special and superior. Such a person is always anxious about his or her shamed and unacceptable "ordinary" humanity and unique individuality. Rage, aloofness, a controlling and demanding attitude, and contempt are often ways adopted for the protection of the narcissistically distorted "good me," the superior self.

The Spurned Child. The spurned child is the abandoned child, the child of neglect. Similar to the shamed child but more deeply disturbed, the spurned child bears the imprint of severe rejection. The pattern of the spurned child tends to manifest itself in two, very different variants, *the hateful child* and *the sad child*. Both subtypes emerge from specific faulty parent-child patterns of coparticipant interaction.

Some parents are overwhelmed or defeated by life's demands and become demoralized and apathetic; consequently they become neglectful, often with an interpersonal attitude that is more depressed and despairing than hostile. In some cases, these parents are too busy with other projects, such as business success or attaining other competitive goals to be bothered with child rearing. This neglect takes many forms, but in all cases parents fail to encourage, assist, guide, and validate their children's needs for tenderness, assistance, and "narcissistic" mirroring from a capable adult, available as an idealized self-other (self-object). In some extreme instances, the child is left, in almost feral condition, to fend for himself or herself, emotionally and sometimes also materially.

This etiology defines the *sad child*: forlorn, lonely, yearning for mirrored approval, often dependent and timid. This child is, in a sense, an emotional orphan. Reactive rage and defensive anger are generally deeply buried, and the manifest diagnostic picture in adulthood, for the milder versions of this pattern, is one of depression, passivity, or, in the terms of an older diagnostic lexicon, neurasthenia, that is, a general sense of weakness and inadequacy. Narcissism here is latent rather than manifest. The depressive patient will evidence covert defensive narcissistic dynamics very much like those described by Walter Bonime (1982a,b) in his long study of the depressive personality.

This pattern of neglect differs from that in the case of the *hateful child*, whose neglect is combined with an extremely harsh parental attitude, one often suffused with rage and possibly accompanied by abuse. This kind of experience may briefly or occasionally emerge in any child-parent relationship. However, in the pattern of the hateful child, it is chronic, intense, and hostile. This pattern fits those children who, according to Sullivan (1953), suffer from a malevolent transformation; the paranoid move from hopefulness and friendliness to a distrustful and hateful need to preemptively strike out at others (to ward off their expected attack). For the hateful child, life is lived with enemies. With this kind of experience, developmental narcissism is dissociated, buried deeply under layers of mistrust and rageful hate. This, of course, is a markedly destructive pattern, both for the person and for those with whom he or she is involved. Pathological narcissism and narcissistic rage are often manifest, but their impact is denied. The child develops an inner sense of self-hatred often covered over by conscious defensive grandiosity and hostility toward others. As adults, these individuals are clinically seen among the sadistically inclined, the psychopathic, the severely paranoid and their symptoms are impulsive acting-out and criminal behavior. Such patients are often incompetent, socially and intellectually, since they have received little guidance or affirmation and certainly very little love, if any at all.

This etiological schematic represents important patterns of parent-child interaction that are significant in the development of narcissistic problems. Three such patterns—the shamed, spoiled, and special children— were initially delineated, as I have discussed elsewhere (Fiscalini 1993). A fourth parent-child pattern—the spurned child and its subtypes, the hateful child and the sad child—is added here. A fifth pattern, the seduced child, the parentally exploited child, could possibly also be included. This would cover the development of narcissism in such psychopathological patterns as the "parentified child," the "Oedipal winner," or those of child abuse, sexual or otherwise. However, I have not examined this pattern thoroughly enough to determine whether it merits inclusion in this etiological schema. Further study is required.

In summary, narcissistic problems may be seen to develop from interpersonal interactions, starting in infancy, that: (a) promote the development of defensive narcissistic ways of being—so-called pathological narcissism; and (b) fail to meet early narcissistic needs for approval that persist in adulthood as repressed aspects of unmet childhood narcissism. These two narcissisms—defensive, or pathological, narcissism and developmental narcissism, the unconscious or preconscious narcissistic aspects of the child's needs for love, dependency, and individuation that are repudiated in the narcissistic developmental process, always coexist. Defensive characterological narcissism can be distinguished from dissociated childhood narcissism by its characteristic insatiability, rigidity, and ruthlessness. Nevertheless, it is not always clear whether some clinical instance of narcissism reflects a wounded childhood need or a requirement of the patient's defensive system, i.e., injured defensive pride. This judgment ultimately can only come from the intensive and intimate work with the patient in coparticipatory therapeutic inquiry, that is, from getting to know the person in his or her singularity.

CHAPTER 8

Coparticipant Inquiry
and Narcissism

Unraveling the psychological meanings and developmental origins of patients' (or analysts') narcissism is a complex and often difficult task. Each analyst and patient represents a complex and variable integral of his or her shamed, spoiled, special, and spurned selves. Consequently, it is seldom clear whether clinical expressions of narcissistic relatedness in the psychoanalytic situation by either patient or analyst represent the transferential or countertransferential living out of dissociated egocentric and "grandiose" developmental needs or the unconscious defensive play of pathological narcissism. If they represent the latter, it is difficult to know whether its origins lie in being indulged, shamed, or shunned.

It is in metapsychological openness—in the freedom to consider new or alternative meanings of their patients' and their own narcissistic behavior and experience—that analysts can creatively grasp the unique meaning of their patients' and their own symptomatology. Only in their recognition that each patient's narcissism is individually patterned and uniquely experienced can analysts envision the possibility of a coparticipant inquiry into the singularity of their patients' and their own narcissism. Analysts' efforts to define the meaning of their patients' narcissistic behavior and experience before inquiring into it openly and in detail invites Procrustean distortion—a surgical fitting of the patient to the analyst's theory. Only in the freedom to understand patients in their developing life rather than "knowing" them beforehand do analysts permit themselves to coinquire *with* the patient into the patient's experience and not merely to inquire *of* the patient about the analyst's view of the patient's behavior.

Rather than applying a metapsychological blueprint of patients' clinical narcissism in the authoritarian manner of many contemporary theorists, analysts may come to a more valid understanding of their patients' psychic uniqueness by openly exploring with them the particular meaning of their narcissism as it emerges and evolves in the psychoanalytic coinquiry. It is a clinical irony that if analysts "know" what they are looking for, they learn only what they already know and nothing more. The opportunity for creation or true discovery is lost, even if security is gained. Paradoxically, it is only when analysts don't "know" what they are looking for that they are open to newness, to the singularity of the other, and to a full and unmeasured knowledge of that other's narcissism. It is only in the mutuality of coparticipant inquiry that patients and analysts allow for an understanding of each other that originates in the immediacy of their clinical work.

Narcissistic countertransference not only emerges from interpersonal tensions within the analytic inquiry but may be implied in the very concept of that inquiry. For example, Otto Kernberg's (1975a) recommended technique for the psychoanalysis of narcissism carries a strong potential for countertransferential shaming of the patient, and Heinz Kohut's (1977, 1984) analytic technique carries a seductive potential for countertransferential spoiling of the patient. More broadly, however, one's very philosophy of inquiry may in itself have a countertransferential structure. I do not mean simply the specific presented theory of treatment but the analyst's fundamental concept of the patient *as a patient*. For example, if analysts arrogate to themselves a position of metapsychological and methodological privilege—if they assume superordinate responsibility and authority for the inquiry—then their coinquiring patients are reduced to the status of children upon whom the analyst imposes his or her preferred metapsychology and methodology. And no matter how benign the analyst or how plausible his or her theory-derived (or theory-driven) understanding, the patient is infantilized, cut off from full participation in a shared inquiry. Inevitably, narcissistic relatedness is countertransferentially reenacted in the analysis. The patient, already stunted in his or her autonomy and individuality, is once again defined by another and is told who he or she is by the analyst. And whether the patient is defined as unmirrored innocent, enraged insatiate, undifferentiated symbiote, or interpersonalized ingratiate matters little. For the fact that the analyst has cast the patient in the narcissistic image of his or her own theory overrides such perspectival differences.

For the *prescriptive analyst,* with his or her hierarchical model of inquiry, interpretation and technique are predetermined by theory rather than emergent in the clinical process. This model of inquiry is inevitably narcissistic: by definition self-centered in its arbitrary foreclosure of coinquiry, grandiose in its assumption of the analyst's procedural and metapsychological superiority, and dismissive of patients' individuality in its authoritarian definition of their psychic experience.

In fact, there are many valid ways to proceed in therapeutic inquiry. Analysts need not maintain, for example, that they must always mirror or allow idealizing, that this is the only right analytic way. Rather, it could be one of many ways, used at different times with different patients and for different reasons. Similarly, analysts need not insist that idealizing is always defensive and that an underlying contemptuous hostility must be interpreted immediately. This, too, could be one of many plausible interpretations, a way to proceed at certain times with certain patients. In other words, analysts may permit themselves to consider the full range of therapeutic possibilities and meanings that emerge spontaneously in analytic interaction with their patients. There is, of course, anxiety in this, for one must make clinical choices and bear personal responsibility for error (of both heart and mind) without the narcissistic cover of theoretical or clinical dogma. In this coparticipant way of working analysts must at some point stand alone, in open relation to their narcissism and their human imperfections. By the same token, however, they also provide for the possibility of standing together *with* their patients, in open relation to their mutual yearning for connection and individuation.

The coparticipant model of inquiry is based on recognizing and respecting patients' inner resources and capability for analytic copartnership. Unlike the infantilizing analyst of authoritarian inquiry, the coparticipant analyst does not reduce the adult in the patient to an analytic child. The coparticipant model of inquiry may, of course, present a countertransference risk that the analyst may "adultify" the patient and expect more of him or her than the patient can cope with. The coparticipatory analyst must be alert to this danger, but while in the authoritarian prescriptive model of inquiry narcissism and implicit dismissiveness of patients' capabilities are built in from the outset, narcissism is not part and parcel of the coparticipatory concept of inquiry except in its misuse.

Coparticipant inquiry calls for open and shared inquiry into both child and adult within both patient and analyst; it acknowledges the regressive and progressive potentials of *both* patient and analyst. Thus, it provides an opportunity for both coparticipants to reach into themselves and to reach out to each other in new, nonnarcissistic ways. In this possibility lies the therapeutic promise of coparticipant inquiry.

NARCISSISM AND COPARTICIPANT INQUIRY

Beyond the analyst's interpretive metapsychology and guiding concept of inquiry there is the question of how he or she specifically works with clinical narcissism as it emerges in the analytic process. For example, what defines the analyst's view of therapeutic action, and how does this affect his or her analytic activity? What defines the analyst's way of approaching and working with "narcissistic" transference and resistance and countertransference and counterresistance? Does the analyst view narcissism as requiring a special technique?

Traditional Freudian analysis—which places the analyst in the role of neutral, ungratifying, and impersonal interpretive surgeon—has premised its therapeutic procedure on the presumed abilities and requirements of the so-called oedipal patient, a presumably healthier and developmentally more advanced patient than the narcissist or borderline character. These latter patients are seen as having a disorder of the primary self, whereas the oedipal patient is seen as suffering primarily from a drive disorder. Traditionally, narcissistic patients have been seen as requiring parametric or modified forms of psychoanalysis—not *real* psychoanalysis, but psychotherapeutic variants of the real thing. Thus, there is a two-tiered system: psychoanalysis for oedipal neuroses, and psychoanalytic psychotherapy for narcissistic patients.

Coparticipant inquiry does not require such a bifurcated concept of treatment (see chapters 1 and 2). This approach to narcissism is characterized by a unique set of therapeutic features which includes, above all, a field conception of narcissistic transference and countertransference, active use of the analyst's self, and detailed and directive as well as free-associative inquiry, emphasis on the analytic interplay of psychic and social reality, in which neither the analyst's nor the patient's subjective "truth" must rule, and a pluralism of interpretive perspectives.

In the coparticipant analysis of narcissism, the analyst is not only a participant observer but also an observed participant. In other words, patients are inevitably participant observers as well as observed participants; they are *coanalysts*, whether or not they are personally, interpersonally, or institutionally constrained from living this out in any particular analysis. This coparticipant concept of shared inquiry acknowledges patients' unique analytic resources and proclivities and allows for a radical individuation of personal interpretive perspectives and methodologies.

Coparticipant psychoanalytic inquiry finds its psychological source in the personal resources of the coinquiring patient and analyst. In contrast to other models of participant inquiry into problems of narcissism, coparticipation emphasizes that patients and analysts shoulder a shared responsibility for analyzing their interpersonal relations and that each coparticipant bears the final, personal responsibility for his or her psychoanalytic self-development.

In a fully coparticipatory inquiry, the clinical analysis of interlocking narcissistic parataxes of patient and analyst—what Wolstein (1959) refers to as transference-countertransference interlocks—may originate with either the patient or the analyst, depending on who in the given moment is most capable of initiating or sustaining such inquiry. From this coparticipatory perspective, patients' analysis of their analysts' narcissistic countertransference in the immediate field of its clinical origin is welcomed as a natural and inevitable expression of analytic curiosity and imagination. In other words, it is welcomed as an expression of patients' individual psychological capacities for experiencing and understanding their own and their analysts' interlocking narcissism.

Every analytic dyad is seen as generating its own unique narcissistic transference-countertransference matrix. Patient and analyst constantly influence one another: inevitably, transference, the patient's distortions of the present as the past, is shaped by countertransference and revealed in it, and countertransference, the analyst's distortion, in turn is shaped by and revealed in the transference. A major technical implication of this coparticipatory view is that understanding the patient's narcissism involves also understanding of the analyst's personality, including his or her narcissistic problems. Countertransference analysis becomes an integral aspect of transference analysis and vice-versa. The shared analysis of countertransference is critical in working with narcissistic patients, particularly since their anxieties and conflicts frequently provoke powerful and disruptive narcissistic countertransference processes.

In the coparticipant analysis of narcissism, the analyst constantly monitors how he or she may be playing out the shaming, spoiling, or shunning countertransferential parent or, conversely, the shamed or spoiled countertransferential child in the narcissistic *introjective transference*. The analyst does not simply focus on what the patient is trying to do, but on what historical interaction is being replayed and on how that is revealed in and related to the analyst's own narcissistic tendencies, as countertransferential parent or countertransferential child.

Coparticipant analysis of narcissism involves the analytic study of patients' anxious interpersonal self (i.e., their narcissistic vulnerabilities and self-personifications) and their defensive self-system functioning (self-object relatedness). This entails an inquiry into the developmental history, analytic vicissitudes, and therapeutic transformation of the patient's self-image.

Coparticipant analysts pay attention to the clinical vicissitudes of the interpersonal self, a concern they share with Kohutian self-psychology. The self-psychological approach, however, focuses exclusively on psychic reality and on a Rogerian-like emphasis on the empathic or client-centered (Rogers 1951) tracking of patients' subjective experience. In contrast, coparticipant inquiry is more inclusive in its detailed inquiry into the interplay of psychic and material reality and in its openness to challenging or questioning the psychic reality of the patient.

Coparticipant analysts realize that narcissistic patients are limited in their ability to tolerate challenges to their subjective perspective and that psychoanalytic work with such patients requires patient and painstaking attention to their narcissistic anxieties. Analysts are mindful that for long periods these patients need the analyst to side empathically with their narcissistic defenses. At the same time, however, analysts who adhere to a coparticipant concept of inquiry believe that active and open coinquiry into patients' as well as their own narcissistic perspectives is essential to analytic growth. Such an approach demands considerable analytic flexibility, emotional openness, and personal maturity on the part of the analyst.

Unlike analysts following other contemporary analytic approaches, coparticipant analysts generally use themselves in their treatment of narcissism. For example, they use more directive and specific questions, allow greater technical freedom to reveal one's own thoughts and feelings, and practice greater self-disclosure. In addition, coparticipant analysts are generally less concerned with an analytic stance of neutrality, particularly in terms of the classical principle of anonymity or the blank screen; they do not hold with the notion of a value-free analyst. Coparticipant analysts also tend to make therapeutic use of countertransference, including freely expressing such analytic experiences.

Another feature of the coparticipant approach to narcissism is its general de-emphasis of regressive technique. Coparticipant analysts, by and large, eschew the concept of technically inducing a regression to a transference neurosis. Most coparticipant analysts believe that regressive aspects of the patient's narcissism will spontaneously emerge, even in an active analytic encounter. In my own clinical experience, I have found that patients' unconscious shamed selves, their persisting unmirrored or disapproved egocentric and naively grandiose childhood yearnings, emerge in the transference from the very beginning of treatment. And patients' transference resistances, the various aspects of their defensive narcissism and narcissistically distorted self-personifications—in other words, their spoiled, special, and spurned (and implicit aspects of their shamed) selves also appear from the very start of an analysis.

An important though not unique characteristic of the coparticipant approach to treatment is its acceptance of the curative role of the "real relationship." Many coparticipant analysts assign an important therapeutic role to the analytic formation of new interpersonal experiences, particularly in the psychoanalytic treatment of more severely disturbed and less verbally accessible patients, such as the more severely narcissistic or borderline person (Fiscalini 1988, 1991).

Coparticipant analysts ascribe great importance to the role of reality in the historical formation and analytic transformation of narcissism. This emphasis on reality is combined, however, with a perspectivistic emphasis and relativistic epistemology—a stance that does not dictate that the analyst's "truth" must rule nor, as Kohut (1984) and others would have it, that the patient's subjective "truth" must rule.

In sum, the coparticipant approach to narcissism is marked by therapeutic open-endedness and flexibility of method. Coparticipant analysts adopt a methodological (and metapsychological) pluralism, deeply convinced that there are many ways to analyze clinical narcissism, not just one right way.

I will now turn to the ideas and work of Kohut and Kernberg. These two theorists are arguably the most influential contemporary Freudian theorists on narcissism. Their different clinical perspectives and contrasting therapeutic sensibilities represent central controversies in the understanding and treatment of narcissistic personalities and problems.

KOHUT'S AND KERNBERG'S APPROACHES TO NARCISSISM: REVIEW AND CRITIQUE

Heinz Kohut (1977, 1984) expanded the interpretive range of mainstream clinical psychoanalysis and broadened its concept of therapeutic action, but he did not seriously challenge accepted principles and procedures of clinical analytic orthodoxy. He remained a neoclassical Freudian. Nevertheless, Kohut's self-psychological approach to narcissism carries a distinctive clinical stamp—a listening perspective that insists on analysts adopting an empathic stance and staying with the patient's subjectivity, while for Kohutians it is some variation of "idealizing," "mirroring," or "twinning" relatedness).

Kohut's aimed above all at fostering the full development and eventual interpretive resolution—via analytic insight—of the narcissistic transferences. Kohut believed that vigorous or systematic interpretation of clinically manifest defensive narcissism would interfere with the emergence of the patient's repressed childhood narcissism, that is, of the dissociated aspects of the shamed, spoiled, special, and spurned child. Kohut focused on patients' shame, loathing, and anxiety about their unconscious or preconscious childhood needs for mirroring and idealizing and on the ease with which, in his opinion, such dissociated transference wishes could be driven underground again after they had emerged. Thus, his technique centered on fostering the clinical emergence of these brittle transferences that were easily shamed and frightened off. Kohut cautioned against the interpretation of narcissistic defenses, advising the analyst to support instead the gradual emergence of the narcissistic transferences by the consistent maintenance of an empathic connection to the unconscious or dissociated mirroring and idealizing longings—unmet and unresolved childhood egocentricity and naive grandiosity—embedded in manifest clinical narcissism.

The analyst, in this view, accepts the transferential mirroring, twining, and idealizing longings of the patient until they are fully mobilized and ready for interpretation—ready, in other words, for optimal analytic disillusionment. The clinical task, as Kohut saw it, is to maintain empathic contact with the unconscious narcissistic aspects of the patient's early needs for love, dependency, and individuation in order to facilitate their full emergence and their optimal disillusionment via interpretive insight. The main effort is to avoid traumatizing the fragile narcissistic longings. Kohut believed that any attention to the social or personal inappropriateness, i.e., immaturity or irrationality, of defensive narcissism or persisting childhood narcissism, including any moralizing about them, would be therapeutically counterproductive.

Kohut acknowledged that it is impossible for analysts to maintain constant empathic contact with their patients. In his opinion, the lapses in empathy provide the opportunity for psychic growth by means of what he called transmuting internalizations. In this process, disruptions in empathy, once they have been corrected and empathy has been restored, are explained and interpreted in all their aspects, including the transferential. If the lapse in empathy can be processed psychically (i.e., it is not too traumatizing), the patient is able to take in the perspective of the analyst and in this way gradually alter his or her narcissism. This process is thought to mimic the normal developmental process of optimal disillusionment. For Kohut, this process and that of interpretive insight form the two means by which analytic self-transformation is brought about.

The striking feature of this approach is not any innovative change in psychoanalytic procedure but its listening perspective—its openness to narcissistic themes and in its prescription for the analyst to always strive to see things from the patient's subjective and narcissistic perspective.

The Kohutian (and post-Kohutian) self-psychological approach to the treatment of narcissism has gained wide popularity and has influenced the clinical approaches of many psychoanalytic practitioners. Its strongest impact, however, has been primarily among mainstream analysts. Self-psychology has brought the study of the interpersonal self within the purview of Freudian psychoanalysis. It has had a lesser impact on British object-relations and American interpersonal-relations analysts, who had already developed notions of the interpersonal self and its treatment.

The popularity of self-psychology is also grounded in the allure of its simplicity. Self-psychology, particularly when understood in simplistic terms, seems to provide a simple diagnostic and therapeutic blueprint—all narcissistic patients suffer from one of two universal narcissistic structures, either a mirroring or idealizing transference (or some variant thereof). This simply has to be identified, and then all other understanding will follow. This formulation is neat and simple and as reductionistic as the orthodox application of the Oedipus template to all pathology and psychology. When understood in more complex terms, however, the idealizing mirroring transferences can be seen to refer to highly complex sets of phenomena whose clinical treatment cannot be reduced to some simple formula or easy-to-use rule book.

Self-psychology also tends to hold a seductive promise that the psychoanalytic process, or even life itself, can be painless and anxiety-free. Self-psychological ideas are often applied in ways that countertransferentially reinforce patients' narcissistic demands and dreams of an interpersonal paradise—life without anxiety.

Passive expectations or hopes of a narcissistic cure—that one can, through the "empathic" intervention or understanding of another, avoid the conflict, uncertainty, and active effort that is inevitable in growth and self-transformation—find a theoretical rationale in Kohut's overly interpersonalized, other-directed account of the human psyche. Like Sullivan, Kohut neglects the domain of the personal self or self-subject relations—the psychic dimension of will, responsibility, individuality, personal agency, and self-generative activity. In other words, Kohut's self-psychology is concerned with the reactive "me," with the individual as socially determined by his or her interpersonal surroundings rather than with the proactive "I," the individual as unique, generative, determining self. This one-sided interpersonal emphasis on self-object relations may countertransferentially abet patients' narcissistic denial of personal agency, their defensive blaming of others, and their neurotic insistence on emotional reparation for losses and injuries suffered in childhood.

Though all patients were once the intended or inadvertent victim of others' anxiety, lack of empathy, or even antipathy, it is also true that all patients are active participants in the neurotic perpetuation of their narcissistic patterns. Kohut's clinical approach overemphasizes the therapeutic role of the interpersonal self-other and thus fails to account sufficiently for the active and interactive role that each patient plays in his or her own development. Although patients are not to blame for their narcissistic problems, they must be held accountable for them.

Therapeutic analysis of patients' narcissistic defensive structures requires, I think, the analyst to initiate eventually a judicious and honest direct appraisal of their harmfulness to themselves and to others in their life. Kohut would argue that such active analytic intervention would be countertherapeutic and would reflect a countertransferential "maturity morality." And indeed, such an approach could reflect the operation of countertransference, but that is not necessarily so. Conversely, one could justly object to Kohut's approach in that it reflects a countertransferential "immaturity morality" in its failure to actively confront patients' self-destructive narcissism. To wait for inadvertent lapses in empathy in order to empathically interpret them to the patient, as Kohut technically advises, is, at the very least, therapeutically inefficient. An even more serious problem with this approach is that it fails to sufficiently address patients' unconscious strivings to grow beyond the confines of their constrictive narcissism and to face themselves. In its "benevolent" authoritarianism and view of the patient as passive, Kohut's clinical approach underestimates patients' inner resources and reserves. And in this, the self-psychological clinical approach courts the danger of becoming superficially supportive, rather than deeply transformative.

One of Kohut's major critics among contemporary Freudians is Otto Kernberg (1975a,b). While Kohut focuses therapeutically on the developmentally arrested or fixated aspects of patients' narcissism, Kernberg targets the pathological developments in narcissism, namely, patients' unconscious or preconscious defensive narcissistic processes. Unlike Kohut, Kernberg aggressively confronts and systematically interprets patients' defensive pathological narcissism, particularly the patients' unconscious rage, contempt, envy, and other hostile ways of devaluing the analyst. Kernberg is sharply critical of what he considers to be Kohut's countertransferential neglect of the negative aspects of the transference. Whereas Kohut prescribes empathic tolerance of developmental and defensive narcissism and cautions against confronting it, Kernberg stresses the importance of precisely this direct confrontation. Kernberg also stresses patients' secondary conflicts over their aggressive "badness," that is, their contempt, rage, and envy. Kernberg maintains that treatment should focus on the narcissistic patient's guilt and fear that his or her hostile aggression will destroy the analyst, provoke the analyst's retaliation, or destroy the patient's own ability to love or receive love, and thus destroy any opportunity for a good and loving relationship. Kohut (1972) does not ignore the patient's aggression but emphasizes the analysis of its anxious underpinnings. Kohut thus analytically targets patients' early narcissistic injuries, that is, their vulnerable interpersonal selves, and he adopts a serene and accepting analytic attitude that is sensitive to the patient's shame and fear. Kernberg, on the other hand, concentrates on patients' defensive narcissism and its destructive and negative impact on the patient and others. Consequently, Kernberg calls for an aggressive and challenging analytic approach to patients' defensive hatred, envy, and contempt. For Kohut, the narcissist is an injured and fallen angel who needs to be rescued and restored; for Kernberg, the narcissist is a pathological devil who must be reformed.

Both Kohut and Kernberg emphasize the importance of interpretation and insight as curative factors; however, Kohut also highlights the curative effect of transmuting internalizations. In other words, he allows for the possibility of emotionally corrective experience. Kernberg, on the other hand, regards interpretation as the only analytically curative instrumentality. Although Kohut's ideas on therapeutic action have been considered heterodox and even unanalytic, I think they are not radical enough. The process of transmuting internalization forms an important, but limited, aspect of a broader curative relational process that I call *living through* (Fiscalini 1988). I believe that working through all narcissistically conflicted patterns of living inevitably involves living them through experientially in new and curatively reconstructive ways in the immediate personal relationship between the patient and analyst (cf. chapter 13). The living through process occurs inadvertently, in both dialectic (i.e., as an integral aspect of the interpretive process) and direct relational (i.e., as direct reconstructive relational experience) forms. This process, particularly in its direct form, is pivotal in the analysis of core, preverbal narcissistic difficulties and deficits.

This process also works in reverse order; that is, the patient may also become a new interpersonal other for the analyst. What takes place relationally between the narcissistic patient and his or her analyst experientially informs both of them about their specific narcissistic difficulties and about new interpersonal and personal possibilities and ways of being; this can directly effect changes in the patient's or analyst's narcissistic character structure.

Although Kohut's and Kernberg's therapeutic sensibilities represent radically different analytic temperaments, divergent clinical emphases, and distinctly different metapsychologies, their visions of narcissism and its treatment are not incompatible. In fact, from a coparticipant perspective, Kohut's and Kernberg's approaches may be seen as complementary. Their differences are not as significant as some insist but show some generally unrecognized similarities. Kohut is generally considered to have defined clinical narcissism as arrested development while Kernberg is believed to have categorized it as pathological development, this distinction does not completely hold true. Instead, each theorist highlights one of these complementary aspects of the problem of narcissism but considers both.

Both Kohut and Kernberg are essentially talking about very early anxious interpersonal relationships in which the child's various strivings for relational intimacy, physical satisfaction, and psychic fulfillment are traumatically rejected, dismissed, or anxiously disapproved of by significant others. In such pathological relatedness, the child's archaic security needs (which are developmentally immature and of a grandiose and idealizing nature) either go unmet or are not met appropriately. Clinical narcissism results when there is severe, prolonged, or repetitive injury to the interpersonal self—that is, to the early narcissistic needs for approval (self-esteem) and consequent substitutive development of self-protective defenses of a narcissistic character (e.g., pathological sense of entitlement, devaluation, idealization, etc.).

Kohut and Kernberg have both made important contributions to the analysis of the interpersonal self within Freudian psychoanalysis. Yet each presents an incomplete and one-sided account of the psychoanalysis of narcissism. Each theorist focuses on an essential aspect of the narcissistic problem but neglects or de-emphasizes those aspects that form the center of the other's theory. A more complete and well-rounded treatment of narcissism requires a comprehensive approach that flexibly considers both arrested (repressed) childhood narcissism (Kohut's emphasis) and pathological developments in it (Kernberg's emphasis) and analytic interplay between the two. Such an approach would correct for the potential therapeutic excesses implicit in Kohut's and Kernberg's one-sided approaches. For example, it would mitigate against the infantilizing and spoiling potential and the danger of analytic masochism implicit in Kohut's approach and against the adultifying and shaming potential and the hazard of analytic sadism implicit in Kernberg's approach.

A final note on Kohut's therapeutic approach is called for here: among the many criticisms that may be leveled at self-psychology, it is justified to question whether Kohut's treatment approach is a solipsistic and narcissistic form of analysis that tends to infantilize the patient and encourage neurotic dependency and thus promotes incomplete or partial as well as protracted or interminable analyses.

NARCISSISM AND COPARTICIPANT INQUIRY REDUX

A pluralistic coparticipant clinical approach focusing on an analytic inquiry into both the interpersonal and personal selves offers a comprehensive therapeutic understanding of narcissism. Such an approach attends to the vital narcissistic dimensions emphasized by both Kohut and Kernberg in an integrated and balanced way. Coparticipant psychoanalysis provides for a flexible blend of therapeutic holding and confrontation, of active work with defenses and respect for patients' vulnerable self-esteem. The coparticipant approach to inquiry, like Kohut's, attends to patients' subjective realities; yet, as noted previously, it also emphasizes the importance of attending to other realities. Thus, coparticipant inquiry is particularly attuned to the interactive and intersubjective properties of the experiential analytic field, certainly more so than most post-Freudian approaches, including those of Kohut and Kernberg. In its therapeutic open-endedness, coparticipant inquiry avoids the one-sided clinical emphases and therapeutic excesses implicit in many contemporary Freudian perspectives.

Coparticipant inquiry represents the flexible application of coparticipatory principles to fit patients' complex therapeutic needs and capacities and analysts' individual ways of working. Therapeutically, coparticipant inquiry into narcissism (as into any other form of human psychic suffering) is a method that gains in clinical richness, power, and flexibility what it may lose in prescriptive certainty.

The narcissistic patient's ability to work analytically is initially limited to a very narrow range of psychoanalytic inquiry. Analysis with these patients requires patient, almost exclusive, attention to subtle issues of self-esteem for prolonged periods of time. The more severely narcissistic the patient, the less he or she is able to tolerate challenges to his or her subjective perspective or pathological narcissism—to his or her defensive needs to idealize others or to be mirrored by them. Narcissistic individuals are similarly limited in their ability to tolerate interpretive interventions or relational interactions that in any way confront them with their dissociated developmental (infantile) grandiosity and egocentricity (repressed shamed experience). This, of course, places limitations on the work. Much of the analytic effort for long stretches of time has to be focused on the self-other dimension of an analysis, on carefully monitoring patients' ability to effectively tolerate inquiry into their narcissistic needs and resistances. The analyst's task of navigating between the dangers of too much and too little anxiety is a very difficult and demanding one that requires considerable self-esteem and centered selfness for a successful coparticipant journey.

Nevertheless, I think that the most therapeutic course is one that emphasizes a highly active and personal engagement of the narcissistic patient. Such interactive engagement requires that the analyst be highly flexible. The analyst must be able to detect and work with sudden and subtle shifts in patients' interpersonal selves (self-esteem) and personal selves (sense of self). Above all, the analyst must have the personal centeredness (relative freedom from personal narcissism) to work nondefensively with the often provocative narcissistic resistances of such patients and with their equally threatening insights into the analyst's own narcissistic problems. Though perhaps less comfortable than other ways of working, an active and challenging approach to the narcissist makes, I think, for optimal analytic progress; it allows for a more penetrating analysis of the patient's personal and interpersonal selves.

As the analyst's narcissism emerges in the countertransference and counterresistance, it further limits the narcissistic patient's already narrow working range. The developmental and defensive narcissisms of patient and analyst may even intersect in such ways that they preclude the possibility of successful work together. That is, their interpersonal working range may become too narrow for effective coparticipant inquiry. The analyst's or patient's analysis of the countertransference may, however, widen the coinquiry enough to begin viable analytic work. In a way, countertransference analysis is the coparticipant analyst's first task with the narcissistic patient. Countertransference analysis by both analyst and patient plays a crucial role in working with narcissistic patients, particularly since their narcissistic anxieties, conflicts, and defenses so often evoke narcissistic countertransference experiences in the coparticipant analytic field.

The dissociated narcissistic yearnings of the patient, whether born of the need for dependency, love, individuation, or assertion, often evoke narcissistic countertransferential desires and anxieties in the analyst. Moreover, patients' defensive narcissism can provoke anxiety in the analyst. Analysts' own defensive narcissism may be wounded by patients' grandiosity and defensive narcissism.

The narcissist can be a trying patient, often ungiving and unforgiving. The analyst may find it emotionally taxing to be treated as inferior, inept, irrelevant, and as subject to rejection or ridicule if he or she risks any expression of analytic affection or assertion. These analytic anxieties may trigger the analyst's retaliatory rage and emotional withdrawal or submissive ingratiation and a defensive bid for vicarious satisfaction of his or her own dissociated spoiled or shamed child (endeavoring to get the patient to live out the analyst's own forbidden childhood desires).

Though countertransference analysis may play a pivotal role in the treatment of narcissism, because of their separation anxiety and defensive need to idealize the analyst, narcissistic patients tend to resist countertransference or counterresistance analysis. This resistance to countertransference analysis may interlock with the analyst's own counterresistance to his or her countertransference analysis. However, the analyst who invites coparticipant inquiry into his or her narcissistic countertransference provides the patient with a therapeutic model of nonnarcissistic relatedness—a living experience with someone who is open to others' ideas, able to ask for help, unafraid of others' evaluations, or able to move forward despite being afraid.

Analysts must work with the many facets of patients' narcissistic defenses, addressing now one and now another aspect of the defensive structure as it plays itself out in the here-and-now transference-counter-transference and in extratransference relationships. The timing, sequential patterning, and method of inquiry into defensive narcissism and developmental narcissism cannot, however, be therapeutically predetermined or prescribed. For a method to be therapeutic, it must emerge from the flow of the coparticipant inquiry.

CHAPTER 9

Narcissistic Dynamics and Coparticipant Therapy
Further Considerations

From the very first moments of their first encounter, analysts and patients interactively live out their central narcissistic hopes, expectations, and problems. Each analytic coparticipant brings to the experiential analytic field his or her unique pattern of dissociated archaic egocentric and grandiose yearnings, idealized personifications of the self and others, and defensive characterology. Both coparticipants bring a unique combination of their shamed, spoiled, special, and shunned selves to the intersubjective analytic field, and the character and course of each analytic pairing develops out of the unique patterning of these selves and their dyadic interplay.

The dialectical relationship between analyst and patient reflects an inner dialectic between the two narcissisms of each coparticipant. These are: (1) repressed childhood narcissism—those dissociated needs for assertion, love, dependency, and individuation that prompt a striving for narcissistic approval, recognition, and acknowledgment; and (2) characterological or pathological narcissism—those defensive behaviors and self-experiences that are shunted into manifestations acceptable to significant others as a result of experiences of anxious shaming or spoiling. Both of these narcissisms inevitably emerge in the transference and countertransference; analytic progress depends largely on the therapeutically valid understanding and experiential living through of these two narcissisms.

It is at times difficult to distinguish between these two narcissisms and separate out the unmirrored from the mismirrored, to tell the clinical residuals and dynamic operations of shamed experience from those of spoiled experience. All people psychologically comprise unique combinations of shamed (deprivation), spoiled (indulgence), and spurned (rejection) experience in relation to a broad array of human needs, and this results in complex patterns of clinical narcissism.

Often shamed experience is embedded within and expressed through spoiled experience. For example, the combination of angry demandingness and claims of narcissistic entitlement, a common narcissistic dynamic, is often revealed to be a narcissistic defense of an individual's fears that he or she doesn't deserve any consideration from others and would not freely be given what is wanted or needed or that he or she would not be able to receive it if offered nor able to stand the frustration or grief of not getting it. Similarly, narcissistic attitudes of entitlement often reveal underlying attitudes of nonentitlement. Patients may consciously or unconsciously claim a right to be angry, reproachful, and entitled to special privileges. Yet, on another level, these same patients transferentially may feel that they have no right or ability to assert their legitimate needs without the defenses of reproach and demand. They may not feel entitled to think of effective ways of presenting their wishes and not free or secure enough to bear the pain and disappointment of frustration or disapproval.

Services or objects demanded are often symbolic of other needs, a metaphor for something else. For example, repressed childhood narcissism—naïve egocentric desire for approval and affirmation of early relational, personal, and sensual needs—are often hidden within pathologic claims. It is important that the analyst not confuse the two, for though it may be difficult to distinguish them, these two narcissisms, developmental and defensive, are not the same thing.

All people carry into adulthood some persisting unmirrored childhood narcissistic longings and needs as well as learned defensive narcissistic behaviors. Though these two forms of narcissism are often clinically intertwined, they are, as just noted, not the same thing. Defensive characterological narcissism and the archaic narcissism of the naively grandiose self are very different narcissisms, with different psychological natures, developmental paths, and dynamic meanings. Archaic developmental narcissism refers to the naturally grandiose or idealizing quality of early human relational, sensual, and personal needs and to the archaic need to be interpersonally approved of in similar egocentric terms. By contrast, defensive self-centeredness derives from the incursive experience of interpersonal shaming and spoiling.

Defensive narcissism tends to be of two types: (1) the covert or "timid" variety with unrealistic idealized self-personifications; this type might be called the grandiose shoulds and oughts of personality and is usually associated with a developmental pattern of shaming experience; and (2) the more overtly entitled, manifestly arrogant, and "loudly demanding" variety, with grandiose self representations, usually associated with the spoiled (particularly the uncivilized) and the spurned child. These patterns of narcissism differ from one another, and both differ profoundly from the archaic narcissism of the egocentric and naively grandiose immature self.

Archaic narcissism reflects the developmentally natural and appropriate egocentric and grandiose or idealizing quality of early human relational, sensual, and personal needs and a like archaic need to be approved of in the developmentally primitive and grandiose terms of the early interpersonal self. This narcissism thus represents the early developmental wish to be cherished, adored, and approved of for early, developmentally appropriate states of being, experiences, and behaviors. If these innocent needs are wounded in childhood, they are later clinically expressed with considerable shame, anxiety, and fear or in symptomatic form (i.e., in defensive narcissistic protective behaviors).

In contrast to archaic narcissism, defensive pathological grandiosity and self-centeredness derives from the incursive and intrusive interpersonal experiences of shaming and spoiling and interferes with the unhampered development of the interpersonal self. These learned narcissisms are the defensive substitutes for the optimal mirroring of the child's reciprocal needs for attachment and autonomy and for limits and expansiveness. Childhood narcissism refers, thus, to the repressed need to be loved in one's imperfect ordinariness and uniqueness; pathological narcissism, in contrast, is marked by the defensive need to be perfect, superior, extraordinary, and special—exempt from the requirements of social interaction. Adult narcissistic demandingness and grandiose entitlement, for example, represent defensive attitudes in which the person's right to demand special treatment is acceptable while his or her right to be independent and self-reliant and to experience and express his or her own thoughts, feelings, and wishes, or to feel that he or she can be given to is repressed or dissociated. The person's need for consideration and respect can be gratified only neurotically and dependently and not independently secured. This narcissism is not an adult form of untamed childhood grandiosity. It is not arrested development but a maldevelopment, a warping of experience and growth. It is narcissism grown defensive due to developmental spoiling and a rejected need for mirroring approval of vital relational, sensual, and personal experiences.

Analysts often find the narcissist's demandingness, arrogant self-centeredness, and externalizing of responsibility irritating and at times even insufferable. These countertransferential feelings are inevitable as the coparticipant analyst finds his or her therapeutic way with this pathology through inquiry and more inquiry, both into the analyst's own counter-transferential narcissism and into the patient's narcissistic resistances. The coparticipant analyst seeks to affirm and validate the patient's developmental narcissism, for example, his or her repressed and shamed self-assertiveness and directness of communication. At the same time, he or she continues to question in depth why the patient holds on to his or her pathological defensive narcissism.

Defensive narcissism has its genesis in: (1) humiliating, sadistic, critical, perfectionistic, demanding, or harsh childhood shaming experience (and the correlate development of unrealistic, grandiose, or narcissistic standards and self-personifications with consequent valuing of an "ideal self" and concomitant devaluation of the actual or real self); (2) spoiling experience, the developmental root of most manifest behavior we call narcissism; and (3) the introjection of shaming parents. Identificatory narcissism often shows up clinically in what may be called the *introjective transference* in which patients, like their shaming or spoiling parents, treat the analyst as they were themselves treated. This identification with the criticizer, humiliator, or devaluator is an often ignored but important source of narcissistic traits in the individual. It forms an important source of information about the developmental experiences of the narcissistic patient when observed in the transference or noted in the analyst's subjective countertransference experience.

The clinical narcissism that the analyst encounters is *not* the indirect or metaphoric expression of repressed early narcissism; it is, rather, the direct expression of the very different form of narcissism that is the defensive outgrowth of shamed and spoiled interpersonal experience. The narcissism of the analytic patient is *not* an adult version of childhood narcissism. This is particularly evident in the defensive narcissism that derives from early spoiling experience and in the identification with the shaming aggressor. The angry, demanding, insistent quality of much of clinical narcissism betrays its anxious underpinnings; these are the marks of the anxious interpersonal interactions and relatedness out of which it is born. The child's narcissistic needs do not share this insistent, angry, rigidly demanded interpersonal quality; they are usually expressed shyly and tentatively. Whereas we tend to characterize defensive narcissism, whether of the shamed or spoiled variety, as childish, the persisting residuals of unmet childhood egocentricity and naive grandiosity have a childlike quality.

How does the analyst differentiate between the spoiled and shamed selves and their different defensive derivatives? Defensive narcissism (particularly that which derives from spoiled experience) often can be distinguished from the narcissism of childlike egocentricity by its characteristic insatiability, rigidity, coerciveness, and general ruthlessness.

Nevertheless, it often remains a complex clinical task to sort out infantile archaic narcissism from its intertwined defensive counterpart and to separate these various defensive forms of narcissism from each other— i.e., to separate out spoiled from shamed experience. As noted earlier, the narcissism of most patients represents a complex combination of their shamed, spoiled, and special selves, and it is often difficult to untangle their complex and intertwined dynamics and etiologies. For example, important aspects of the patient's defensiveness, such as certain entitlement attitudes or grandiose ideas, derived from shamed or spoiled experience may themselves be repressed, and they may symptomatically mimic early developmental forms of narcissism. The resulting confusion complicates clinical understanding of the patient. The patient, in other words, may be fearful and anxious about working through both shameful and "shameless" forms of defensive narcissism as well as shamed aspects of early living.

For each patient (and analyst) the developmental origin and dynamic meaning of both their archaic narcissism and their various substitutive narcissisms are uniquely patterned. The patient's narcissism and its dynamic complexities cannot be predetermined beforehand by metapsychological fiat, with the analyst assuming interpretive supremacy. Nor can it be truly discovered by therapeutic authoritarianism, in which the analyst assumes a superior role in inquiry. The complex and unique meaning of each patient's narcissism can be most fully understood and therapeutically lived through in a coparticipant analytic inquiry in which both patient and analyst collaboratively inquire into the patient's narcissistic processes as they interact with those of the analyst.

Despite the complexities and difficulties of differentiating the two narcissisms, analytic progress requires that the analyst and patient live through and understand the patient's and to some extent also the analyst's archaic narcissism and the various defensive forms of narcissism. The patient's unconscious shamed self—the persisting unmirrored egocentric and naively grandiose yearnings of childhood—will emerge in transactions in the transference from the very beginning of treatment. The same is true for the patient's transference resistance—his or her defensive narcissism.

If analysts consistently fail to distinguish between archaic narcissism and its defensive substitutes, mistaking the shamed child for the spoiled child (or vice-versa), they will analytically repeat the original *narcissistic trauma*. This will lead to a traumatic, rather than transmuting, internalization of analytic experience and result in either traumatic disillusionment or traumatic illusionment. If signs of the patient's archaic narcissism are misinterpreted as those of defensive narcissism, the original early shaming experience, or *adultilizing*, of the patient will be reenacted in the analysis. This traumatic failure to empathically mirror the patient's early egocentricity and naive grandiosity will result in *traumatic disillusionment*, rather than in a developmentally healthy and interpersonally sensitive disillusionment. Conversely, if defensive narcissism is countertransferentially mistaken for childlike egocentricity, there will be an analytic reinforcement and repetition of spoiling experience, a countertransference reinforcement of the uncivilized, infantilized, or special child, leading to *traumatic illusionment*—a failure to help the patient become more realistic and resourceful.

By focusing on the unmirrored aspects of the patient's functioning, Kohut neglected working actively enough with the patient's *mismirrored narcissism*. Both infantile narcissism and the developmental need for increasing independence, separateness, and maturity must be addressed in therapy.

Pathological claims and attitudes of entitlement, demands for special treatment, and self-centered disregard of others should be understood for what they are: the defensive result of spoiled experience, the developmental residual of the uncivilized and infantilized selves. Some narcissistic patients defensively interpret their interpersonal problems with others as stemming from their masochism when, in fact, their problems actually originate in their grandiose narcissistic expectations and demands. These patients' difficulties with self-acceptance lead to compensatory strivings for narcissistic ascendance and constant attempts to extract admiration, approval, and subservience from others.

Because of their low self-esteem and immaturity, these patients tend to attract and associate with people who have serious psychological problems. Initially enthralled with their self-object choices, these narcissists eventually become disappointed with their "love" choices and defensively consider themselves the masochistic victims of their partners' unreasonableness. Acutely sensitive to their partners' narcissism, they selectively ignore the unreasonableness of their own expectations and demands and the narcissistic character of their object choice. They refuse to accept their partners for the imperfect humans that we all are. Moreover, these patients' irrational dependency and narcissistic neediness and insecurity inhibits an appropriate assertiveness regarding their partner's actual interpersonal disjunctiveness and defensiveness. These themes are expressed and lived out in the transference-countertransference relationship.

Though the partners of the narcissist usually have very real problems, they often manifest genuine capacities for closeness and caring. Unfortunately, however, the mutual insecurities of the narcissist and his or her partner often provoke reciprocal anxieties, and their mutual defensiveness is continuously reinforced; as a result any moves toward shared satisfaction or intimacy are aborted. All too often, complaining narcissistic patients focus on their partner's limitations (real or imagined) and overlook their own and their partners' actual capacity for intimacy. Instead, they berate their partners for their inability to gratify their impossible narcissistic demands and thus remain unloving and unloved.

A common and important underlying dynamic in these problematic narcissistic interpersonal relations is the narcissistic patient's repudiation and fear of autonomy. That is, the narcissistic individual defensively arrogates all interpersonal and relational power and personal responsibility to the other and demands to be taken care of and given special status. The other-directed narcissist, preoccupied with gaining the approval of others, often irrationally fears that achieving or even striving for psychological autonomy would inevitably result in a frightening disconnection and isolation from others rather than in a centered and more secure and mature form of relatedness.

Narcissistic patients need to become more aware, both through interpretation and experience, that they only esteem themselves on narcissistic grounds—that they don't value themselves as they actually are, but only when they can feel special or superior. Narcissists cannot value themselves in their uniqueness, nor can they freely accept their separateness; instead, they strive defensively for self-centered symbiosis and a sense of specialness. This problem must be empathically and repetitively lived through and interpreted. Both the narcissist's chronically low self-esteem and his or her substitutive narcissistic self-expectations and behaviors must be worked through in coparticipant inquiry. The resolution of the patient's narcissism requires both interpretive insight and experiential living through of the patient's pathological narcissistic self-inflation and narcissistic defenses *and* the underlying unmet mirroring or idealizing needs, the anxious "not me" experience. Narcissistic "good me" defensiveness must be worked through and relinquished; it must be transformed, as it were, into a no longer needed "bad me"—to be replaced by previously repressed "not me" aspects of the true self that are now reintegrated as a new, non-narcissistic "good me." This is often a lengthy process.

Unlike the noisy narcissist with his or her shameless overt defensive arrogance, the timid narcissist experiences the grandiose striving for narcissistic gratification as shameful. Thus, for timid narcissists the analysis of resistance (defensiveness) is a two-step process. Since they experience their defensive grandiosity as shameful and thus deny (repress) it, it must be brought to awareness before it can be worked through and resolved.

For the timid narcissist, the analysis of the resistance to the awareness of resistance (in other words, the analysis of the patient's defensiveness of defensiveness) must precede the analysis of the resistance to the awareness of transference, of repressed need. This two-step process is equally necessary for the analysis of counterresistance (the analyst's resistance) to the awareness (and resolution) of counterresistance. The coparticipant analyst, to the extent he or she is free of narcissism, encourages the patient to participate in a coinquiry into their shared and multileveled resistance-counterresistance matrix. In any event, patients' awareness of their defensive narcissism is a prerequisite for coinquiry into the nature of transference residuals of the shamed need for mirroring approval of the activity of the relational, sensual, and personal selves.

Narcissistic patients reject those aspects of their analysts' personalities that they reject in themselves, the same ones that were originally rejected by the patients' caretakers. Because of the nature of their self-rejection, narcissistic patients are very hard on the analyst's self-esteem. Contemptuous of their own human ordinariness and imperfections, narcissistic patients are rejecting of the analyst's ordinariness and imperfections. Such patients also eschew a sense of the analyst and themselves as unique and separate individuals.

Narcissistic patients are characteristically both rejecting and demanding. The analyst is seen as worthless yet able to satisfy the patient's demands. Obviously, this coparticipant situation is difficult for analysts and can provoke defensiveness and processes of self-rejection in them. Therapeutic coparticipant inquiry into these swirling defensive transferential and countertransferential currents requires that the analyst has a robust interpersonal self and a strong self-esteem. The analyst also needs ready access to his or her personal self, to his or her creative clinical powers and unique sense of individuality. Only with such resources can the devaluing be weathered and the therapeutic coinquiry be advanced into that defensive maelstrom of narcissistic contempt and arrogance. This coparticipant inquiry is undertaken in the search for the patient's (and the analyst's own) unmet and repressed needs for love, sensual satisfaction, and self-fulfillment.

The curative coparticipant process depends significantly on analysts' ability to correct their countertransference misappraisals of their patients' narcissism and on their ability to be open to signs of their countertransferential impact when it manifests itself in patients' reactive depression, anxiety, or mania.

The countertransferential shaming or spoiling of a patient is, of course, rooted ultimately in the analyst's own personal narcissism, though, as argued earlier, this narcissism may be institutionalized in certain concepts of inquiry or theories of psychopathology, for example, in the *infantilizing* and *adultilizing* potentialities that are implicit in the theories and therapeutic approaches of Kohut (1971, 1977, 1984) and Kernberg (1975a,b). (Adultilization and infantilization are further discussed in chapter 13.)

Countertransference distortions are inevitable. They may even be therapeutically useful, and they are not necessarily harmful if corrected. In other words, it is inevitable that the analyst will make mistakes of perception and intervention. It is imperative, however, that these be identified and, when possible, analyzed and rectified in the coparticipant inquiry. This facilitates and allows patients to gain therapeutic self-understanding and to live through their early unmet narcissistic needs, archaic narcissistic anxieties, and maladaptive narcissistic defensiveness in therapeutically reconstructive ways. All this must be lived through and empathically understood to provide for the fuller living out of stunted early needs and to allow new ones to grow from them.

The successful analytic treatment of narcissism requires a flexible deployment of attention to both unmet childhood egocentric needs and defensive grandiosity and self-centeredness as now one and now another of these dimensions of the patient's (and analyst's) narcissism play themselves out in the coparticipant analytic interaction and coinquiry.

Demandingness and a grandiose sense of entitlement are frequently observed narcissistic symptoms. These attitudes often provoke anger in analysts who work with narcissistic patients and in patients who work with narcissistic analysts. It is not the exorbitant wishes of the narcissistic individual that arouses the reactive anger in others, but rather their insistence that others should comply with their wishes. The analyst's (and patient's) reactive and self-protective (defensive) anger has multiple roots, including the provocation of his or her latent grandiosity, the irrational belief that one should be perfect, omnipotent, and omniscient. This represents analysts' failure to accept their own imperfections and limitations. The most effective antidote to another's narcissism is to outgrow one's own narcissistic defensive needs and to develop a mature respect for one's own uniqueness (as opposed to specialness), separateness (as opposed to symbiosis), and limitations (as opposed to grandiosity). In this way, by largely overcoming narcissism in oneself, one inevitably frees oneself of the narcissistic demands of others. One can, then, chart one's own course, whether in the coparticipant field of psychoanalysis or in the coparticipant fields of everyday life.

Another important narcissistic dynamic is the fear of dependency and influence. Narcissistic patients often feel shame about *real or true dependency* yet shamelessly insist on immediate gratification of defensively learned *neurotic dependency.* In other words, they have serious difficulty in experiencing and expressing true, developmentally arrested, needs for support, help, guidance, and supportive tenderness but, paradoxically, insist on gaining defensively required "babying." This defensive dynamic serves to avoid fears of possible rejection of the need for tenderness. This dynamic, historically learned in indulged or spoiled experience, also serves to defend against the frustration of the desire for autonomy.

Both dependencies, developmental and defensive, may include immature dependency, but they spring from different sources—arrested early interpersonal need in the one case and pathologically developed defense in the other. These two kinds of dependency have different meanings and require different therapeutic relatedness. The narcissistic patient is characteristically both defensively dependent and defensively independent (counterdependent) and, simultaneously, phobic of true dependency and true independence (autonomy). Thus the patient requires *both* optimal gratification of shamed need and optimal frustration of shameless or spoiled defensive need.

Narcissistic individuals, often characterized as selfish and self-serving, have great difficulty with the give-and-take of ordinary social interactions. In their ceaseless search for reflected approval, narcissistically inclined people are focused on securing affirmation and admiration from others. Given their developmental immaturity, they are unable to genuinely consider others' needs or wishes.

Like all immature people, narcissists usually give in order to get—to get approval, to ingratiate themselves, to impress others, or to manipulate them. However, those who are more mature and can identify with others, give simply because it feels good to give; the giving is experienced as though one were giving to oneself. This, of course, defines altruism and generosity, and it represents that advanced stage of interpersonal development that Sullivan called chumship or love and that Freudian analysts refer to as the genital character.

Feeling oneself to be an acceptable member of the human race, one gives freely of one's attention, time, and talents to oneself and to others. In contrast to insecure narcissistic bids for "self-object" approval, this form of giving comes from one's love of oneself and others. This generosity, and the sense of self-worth it presupposes, is rare in our psychologically immature, pathologically competitive, and interpersonally insecure world, but it does exist. And through the wider dissemination of psychoanalysis, particularly in its coparticipant forms, it may proliferate.

Analysts' narcissistic anxieties may lead to an overly aggressive analytic approach; for example, the analyst may countertransferentially respond to his or her patient's narcissistic dependency and "selfish" demands for perfect understanding by becoming excessively demanding and exhorting the patient to be more mature. This is good advice but therapeutically counterproductive. In this way, the analyst falls back on what

Kohut called a reality morality, a countertransferential dismissiveness of the patient's anxiety and immaturity. If the patient could simply be mature—through an effort of will—he or she would. What patients need is a nonjudgmental coinquiry into why and how they unconsciously refuse to move forward or are unable to do so.

Narcissistic countertransference may also express itself in a therapeutic timidity or in an analytic approach that is overly supportive. Analysts may defensively deal with their inability to accept their therapeutic imperfections or limitations by denying them and unconsciously insisting on playing out the role of the omnipotent and omniscient "big Daddy" or "good Momma" analyst who can take care of everything and satisfy what, in fact, may be insatiable demands (Tenzer 1987).

An undue preoccupation with the vicissitudes of the interpersonal self and an excessively supportive approach that insists on maintaining empathy with patients' narcissism runs the therapeutic risk of reinforcing their childhood experiences of being infantilized and spoiled, and it ignores the patient's developmental needs to progress beyond their childhood narcissistic fixations. The analyst's empathy with the patient's interpersonal self—his or her representational self—should be balanced by empathy with the patient's unconscious personal, relational, and sensual selves and his or her developmental strivings toward personal (psychic) fulfillment, relational intimacy, and sensual (physical) satisfaction (Fiscalini 1991). An excessive focus on empathy with patients' shamed experience runs the risk of not being challenging enough and of leading patient's to despair of ever being able to grow psychologically.

A prevalent issue in the analysis of narcissism is the defensive dynamic of controllingness. Many an analysis founders on this problem. Though this problem is not unique to the treatment of narcissism, it is exacerbated in analytic work with narcissistic patients. Analysts are often hoist on their own grandiose petards when they strive to overcome their patients' stubborn and often impervious resistances. Unresolved omnipotent and omniscient strivings in analysts often prove to be a fertile ground for countertransference provocation by narcissistic patients. Idealizing aspects of the transference, for example, may lull analysts into analytic complacency by neurotically gratifying the analyst's defensive grandiosity.

The psychoanalysis of narcissism always involves the narcissistic patient's imperative need to work through his or her self-defeating defensive narcissistic patterns of living and to live through and resolve his or her early narcissistic anxieties. The analysis of narcissism, thus, always requires a flexible attention to defensive and infantile narcissism, to the developmental need for limitless acceptance and acceptable limits, to spoiling and shaming, to the patient's subjective perspective and the analyst's alternatives, to the need for security and for growth. In other words, the analyst must keep in mind both the interpersonal and the personal self as they emerge in the narcissistic transference-countertransference matrix. And the same is true for the coparticipant patient.

The analytic formation of new interpersonal experience is crucial in the treatment of narcissistic patients. The curative action of therapy with narcissistic patients is centered in the living of a nonnarcissistic relationship. Nonnarcissistic attitudes comprise an integral aspect of a broader and more inclusive curative relational process that I call the *living through process* (Fiscalini 1988; see also chapter 13). I believe that the working through of all narcissistically arrested patterns of living inevitably involves the experiential living through of these patterns in new and curatively reconstructive ways in the immediate personal relationship between patient and analyst.

From a coparticipant perspective this process also works in the other direction; that is, the patient may become a new interpersonal other for the analyst, hence relationally curative for the analyst's unresolved narcissism. What takes place relationally between the narcissistic patient and his or her analyst experientially informs both of them about their specific narcissistic difficulties and about new interpersonal and personal possibilities and ways of being. Over time this directly effects changes in the patient's *or analyst's* narcissistic character structure.

The working through of clinical narcissism in both its developmental and defensive aspects rests upon analysts' ability to authentically live through significant dimensions of their patients' *and their own* narcissism in interpersonally new and different ways. It is in this living through process that patients develop the deep, *emotional* conviction that new and nonnarcissistic ways of living are not only preferable, but possible—that one can, in fact, move psychologically from the despair of constrictive self-centeredness to the hopefulness of expansive, centered selfness and the ability to think, feel, and act for oneself.

PART FOUR

EXPLORATIONS IN THERAPY

CHAPTER 10

Openness to Singularity
Facilitating Aliveness in Psychoanalysis

Psychological aliveness, as both theme and experience of inquiry, is a central concern for all analysts. As a central theme in psychoanalytic treatment, therapeutic aliveness calls to mind such processes and experiences as creation, exploration, play, wonder, and discovery. Psychoanalysis is fundamentally about life, about living it creatively and passionately and, of course, reflectively. It is, after all, the living of life, the psychological working through of irrational difficulties in living, and the radical transformation and deepening of our living that makes up the psychoanalytic agenda. And for those of us who practice it, psychoanalysis is our life's work and our way of making a living.

But what of aliveness as experience of psychoanalytic inquiry? The problem of creating psychoanalytic aliveness, an alive and vital inquiry, confronts us all. Whether our inquiry is alive or not is a crucial dimension of our work we must never neglect.

In this chapter, I consider an essential aspect of coparticipant inquiry and the facilitation of analytic aliveness I call *openness to singularity*. This is not an attempt to advise various methods on how to quicken inquiry but an effort to explore a crucial dimension of analytic relatedness which bears significantly on the facilitation of analytic depth and creativity, that is, of aliveness in the psychoanalytic process.

The question of what is essential in keeping a psychoanalytic coinquiry moving, alive, or going forward rests upon the more basic question of what we mean by an alive inquiry. On this point, analysts often differ. What one analyst calls aliveness may be what another would label wild analysis; one analyst's activity may be what another would consider acting out, and so on. Such differences may be irreconcilable since they are grounded in personal preference and prejudice and theoretical loyalty. A definition satisfactory to all may not be possible. Nevertheless, I think it is possible to provide a broad definition of psychoanalytic aliveness that would satisfy most, if not all, analysts, coparticipant or not.

Any concept of psychoanalytic aliveness requires that we first distinguish between an alive analytic inquiry and a lively one. An alive analytic process may or may not be a lively experience, and conversely a subjectively lively experience may or may not reflect aliveness in the analytic process itself. A subjectively felt quality of vibrancy, vividness, movement, intensity, or depth in analytic interaction usually, perhaps always, signals alive currents in the coparticipant psychoanalytic enterprise. It may, however, simply reflect a defensive, though emotionally vivid, relatedness. Consider, for example, the analytic liveliness that an all too measured obsessional analyst may feel in the presence of a coquettish and charming hysteric, the intellectualized analytic soaring of kindred ideational spirits, the sado-masochistic excitement of a subtle but destructive analytic power relationship, the narcissistic delights of two self-absorbed analytic partners, and similar analytic constellations. Rather than pointing to an alive inquiry in the coparticipant analytic encounter, such analytically lively sparks may indicate the opposite—conflictual energy going nowhere, all sparks and no fire. Such situations may represent interactional sparks that, if harnessed analytically (such as in "here and now" transference-countertransference analysis), may fuel an alive coparticipant inquiry.

Similarly, the subjective experience of analytic deadness—of dullness, boredom, lethargy, lack of interest, futility, or a sense of going nowhere—generally reflects some defensive deadening of the analytic process, some resistive or counterresistive effort to stifle, derail, or otherwise block a progressively broadening and deepening contact and growing intimacy between analyst and patient. However, this is not always the case. There may be growth and movement in a seemingly static analysis, but it may be subliminal, in a state of incubation, as it were. Analytic life may proceed, quietly and unnoted, under the protective cover of seeming lifelessness.

Basically, in its simplest and broadest sense, aliveness in the psychoanalytic situation describes the progressively deepening, broadening, and increasingly therapeutic movement of a psychoanalytic coinquiry. In practice this means that the coparticipant inquiry moves continuously toward increasingly transforming inquiry into transference and countertransference, resistance and counterresistance, anxiety and counteranxiety, and patients' and analysts' centeredness. Aliveness in psychoanalytic coinquiry is evident in an expanding mutual inquiry into both patients' and analysts' personal and interpersonal selves. This may show itself in significant shifts in the patient's or analyst's ways of being and relating; deeply personal changes, even if unarticulated, not consolidated, or in a state of flux; a focused grappling with central problems; discovery of previously unknown connections between formerly disparate aspects of living. Psychoanalytic aliveness may also manifest in a subjective sense of being enhanced, empowered, or freed as evidenced in both everyday living and in analytic responsivity; confrontation of inadequate and inappropriate patterns of living; the emergence of new data and the generation of new perspectives on older data, and the emergence of new memories. Further, aliveness in psychoanalysis is evidenced in the resolution, however partial, of long-interfering characterological inadequacies; the emergence of new feelings, or new strength of feelings or new connections between them; the development of greater introspectiveness and analytic curiosity, and the ability to shoulder more of the analytic inquiry; the emergence of new analytic themes; and so on. In short, an alive inquiry is one characterized by expansion, flow, generativity, and growth. And from a coparticipant perspective, it inevitably involves an analytic reciprocity. That is, an alive coinquiry requires psychic aliveness in *both* coparticipants.

Though psychic aliveness may characterize the coparticipants' usual level of relatedness, at any given point in an analysis either the analyst or the patient may be more alive in his or her analytic coparticipation. For an analysis to be fully alive and transformative, *both* coparticipants must be fully awake, as Fromm might put it. Thus the analyst's responsibility is not only to develop such aliveness in himself or herself but also to foster or encourage its development in his or her patient, in general and in the specific analytic moment.

By implication, lack of aliveness in inquiry is characterized by analytic constriction, blockage, sterility, and stasis. It also manifests itself in endless repetition of analytic themes without discernible changes of any sort; patients' barren dream (and associational) life; lack of change in the patient (or analyst), whether in the transference or in everyday life; failure to develop new perspectives and analytic material. The lack of aliveness in inquiry also manifests itself in prolonged and fruitless silences (or conversely, logorrhea); continued avoidance of central problem areas; refusal to acknowledge or inquire into transferential or resistant (and countertransferential and counterresistant) analytic coparticipation; and so on.

Aliveness in an analysis depends, of course, on a multiplicity of factors and ultimately on the contributions of *both* participants and their compatibility. The analyst facilitates movement or aliveness in the psychoanalytic situation not by the application of specific prescribed techniques but by developing a set of capacities or attitudes that lead to specific interventions, whether by analyst or patient.

Aliveness in inquiry, the moving forward or deepening and broadening of inquiry, depends on a combination of factors that can be subsumed under the general rubric of analytic assistance or facilitation of analytic process. I am referring here to that complex of psychic processes, behaviors, and experiences that promote the analytic inquiry.

Analytic assistance or facilitation thus comprises everything the analyst and patient do that moves coparticipant analysis forward. This includes all "within" the analyst or patient that move him or her toward the other and into an increasingly deeper and more intimate inquiry. Facilitation may be thought of as an essential parameter of analytic inquiry, standing in direct and symmetrical contrast to resistance and counterresistance, and joining transference and countertransference, anxiety, and selfness as a defining characteristic or dimension of psychoanalytic inquiry.

OPENNESS TO SINGULARITY

One group of interrelated psychological capacities in particular comprises a central dimension of analytic facilitation. This group of therapeutic processes collectively form an orientation or attitude toward inquiry that may be called *openness to singularity*, defined briefly as an *attitude of openness to the uniqueness and individuality or specificity of any particular person, process, or analytic moment*. Openness to their singular coparticipatory experiences is essential for both analyst and patient, and it constitutes an instrumental part of an analyst's ability to keep an analysis alive.

The capacities and attitudes that comprise openness to singularity may also be considered parts of play, aspects of creativity, or dynamic features of personal autonomy and interpersonal maturity. These capacities and attitudes are embedded in and operate through a complex of such essential analytic processes as empathic relatedness, personal warmth, emotional sensitivity, and clinical imaginativeness and judgment.

The psychological capacities and qualities that comprise *openness to singularity* are:

therapeutic curiosity;
clinical innocence (the capacity for surprise);
solitariness (the capacity to be alone);
fallibility (the ability to be wrong); and
spontaneity.

Curiosity

All inquiry begins with *curiosity*; indeed, curiosity about the human psyche, conscious and unconscious, is the root of all psychoanalytic inquiry and coinquiry. Without the patient's and analyst's active curiosity the entire coparticipant psychoanalytic enterprise withers and dies. To be therapeutic, this curiosity must be directed toward the singular and specific.

Optimally, this curiosity is turned evenly toward the singularity of the self, that of the other, and the immediate interpersonal relatedness of analyst and patient in the analytic "here and now." It should not be focused exclusively on the psychic life of the patient, but must also include the analyst's own intersubjective and personally unique experience in the relationship with the patient.

Although the drive to explore the many dimensions of the human psyche may lead to the forming of interpretive pattern, inferential order, or symbolic abstraction, it begins in wonder about the mystery of the particular, in the desire to grasp singularity, to know the unique person one is encountering. It is this very uniqueness, the "strangeness" and "otherness" of another person or process that grips our imagination and prompts our efforts at understanding and symbolizing it. The universal is born in the singular. It is interesting to note that one of the archaic meanings of the term curiosity is "being done with painstaking accuracy or attention to detail." The etymological root of curiosity turns out to be the same as that of the word cure, the Latin *cura* or care, suggesting perhaps the intimate therapeutic relation between these processes.

The therapeutic curiosity of the analyst manifests itself not simply in an exploratory interest in the specifics of the patient's narratives and, as Sullivan (1953) would have us observe, the omissions, gaps, or what is *not* in patients' reports of their everyday life experience—in the telling discontinuities in their narratives. Analytic curiosity extends most crucially into the singularity of the analyst's relatedness to his or her patient, provoking the analyst's inquiry into such particulars as: why does this patient say or do *this* (but not *that*) to and with me at *this* time in *this* way. And similarly, why do I feel, think, do, or say *this* with him or her, in *this* unique way at *this* time, and so on, in an ever-expanding and deepening coinquiry. Often, curiosity manifests itself in the consideration of alternatives, in reflecting on why some other *that* instead of *this* is not taking place.

To be effective in analysis, the analyst's curiosity must reach further than the usual inquiry into the interpersonal intimacy (or lack thereof) of analyst and patient, to the interpersonally unique or the "me-you." It must extend into the personal relationship each coparticipant has with himself or herself, into the personally unique, the "me-I," or the first -personal, as Wolstein would call this dimension of the psyche.

The analyst's capacity to be curious about the patient and himself or herself is analytically necessary to maintain an alive inquiry, and this curiosity also stimulates the development and expression of this capacity in the patient. All too often, patients' capacities for wonder, curiosity, and imaginative inquiry have lain fallow, undeveloped, and untutored and perhaps have even been repressed, thwarted, or forbidden.

Cultural homilies such as "curiosity killed the cat" or cultural derogations such as "being too nosy" reflect our culture's proscription of alive wonder and interest in the singularity of one's self and that of others. The psychological curiosity that so typifies and energizes the infant's and child's fascination with the actions and interactions of others and themselves (and later, of their subjective states) all too frequently atrophies or disappears from the neglect, disapproval, or prohibition by significant others.

Interestingly, psychology and psychoanalysis are strikingly incurious about curiosity. The work of Ernest Schachtel and, more recently, that of D. B. Stern are notable exceptions.[1] Nevertheless, there is relatively little written directly on the subject. Why? This lack of interest in curiosity may be due to the fact that it is generally taken for granted as a given, a part of human nature, essential in our particular work (or in life, for that matter)that needs no explanation or exploration? The clinical truth, however, is that both patient and analyst often lack curiosity. Both Freud and Sullivan, originators of perhaps the two most ambitious efforts at analytically comprehending the human psyche, curiously enough fail to provide any construct for understanding this human drive in its own terms. For Freud, all forms of curiosity are derivative scoptophilia or sublimated primal voyeurism. And Sullivan, that most clinically curious of therapists, developed no theory explaining curiosity. Thus, the study of curiosity has been left primarily to the humanistic psychologists, such as Maslow, experimentalists like Berlyne, and developmental researchers and theorists.

Nevertheless, curiosity is at the core of the process that fires the psychoanalytic imagination and fuels the successful coparticipant inquiry. One can observe over and over again how all good analytic work reveals therapeutic curiosity at its core. We can all appreciate the quality of open curiosity that so consistently characterizes that published clinical work we view as most alive. Vignettes illustrating the central role of curiosity in psychoanalytic inquiry can be found in the work of Levenson (1972), Singer (1965), Wolstein (1959, 1988), and Zucker (1967), among others.

Clinical Innocence: The Capacity for Surprise

An integral part of curiosity, the capacity for clinical innocence is by and large similar to what Arieti (1976) called "gullibility,"or the "willingness to suspend disbelief" (p. 377), an attitude he considered essential for creativity. Clinical innocence here means the ability to be surprised, suspend judgment, to follow an exploratory path of inquiry that is uncertain, ambiguous, or unfamiliar. Clinical innocence is a state of openness that many analysts, given their predominately obsessive or schizoid character structures, find difficult to maintain, especially since such a premium is put on formulating experience and achieving analytic order and predictability.

Clinical innocence is the ability, in Schachtel's (1959) term, to disembed oneself from contextual familiarity and to open oneself to the unfamiliar. It is the capacity to see the patient in his or her own unique terms. It is closely related to both empathy and sympathy. Clinical innocence and the capacity for surprise allow the analyst to see the patient without prejudice and preconceived notions. In a sense, clinical innocence may be at the heart of true analytic neutrality, which is based on the personal autonomy and interpersonal maturity of the analyst, as opposed to the conventional concept of neutrality as enforced impersonality. Bion's oft-noted comment that analysts must see the patient with fresh eyes, without memory or desire, captures much of what I mean by clinical innocence. This innocence and analytic attitude of childlike openness is the clinical form of the childlike naivete that Maslow (1971), following Santayana, calls a second innocence or second naivete. This attitude shares much with what Schachtel calls the allocentric attitude and describes as

> one of profound interest in the object, and complete openness and receptivity toward it, a full turning toward the object which makes possible the direct encounter with it and not merely a quick registration of its familiar features according to ready labels. The essential qualities of the interest, the turning toward, the object are its totality and affirmativeness. The totality of interest refers both to the object in which the perceiver is interested and to the act of interest. The interest concerns the whole object, not merely a partial aspect of it; and the perceiver turns toward the object with his entire being, his whole personality, i.e., fully, not just with part of himself. The act of interest is total and it concerns the totality of its object. Indeed, one is the function of the other. (1959, pp. 220–221)

Freud also recommended an attitude of analytic openness that may be called one of innocence. Unfortunately, he did not always follow his own good advice:

> The most successful cases are those in which one proceeds, as it were, without any purpose in view, allows oneself to be taken by surprise by any new turn in them, and always meets them with an open mind, free from any presuppositions. (1912b, p. 327)

Freud's comments about openness to the new or unexpected in the analytic other—like Schachtel's concept of world-openness—holds equally true for the analyst's relationship to his or her own individuality and self-ness. As Theodore Reik (1933/1976) emphasized long ago, psychoanalytic aliveness requires not only openness to the other but also a complementary openness to one's own inner world. As Reik explains,

> It is . . . astonishing to see how often an analyst thinks it enough to follow with uniform attentiveness the associations of the analysand. But listening is not enough; he must hear what the patient says, but, at the same time, he must hear what his own inner voice says, and he must have the courage to understand it, even if the connections do not become plain to him until much later. Of course, he need not say what comes into his mind nor surrender himself passively to it, but he must learn to pay attention to it and keep hold of it. He must have the courage to understand; but also he must have the courage not to understand what his own need for logical connections, his common sense and his conscious knowledge try to thrust upon him. He must have the courage not to understand, even when analytic theory suggests to him certain expectations, when he seems to be going upon conscious psychological knowledge. (p. 381)

Reik continues:

> The analyst's attitude . . . will be that of St. Joan in Bernard Shaw's play, when she is told that the Church prescribes this and that: "But my voices do not tell me so." The technique of analysis cannot be learnt in the abstract: it can only be won from living experience. The courage to understand and the courage not to understand—these are not intellectual qualities, but a matter of character, an expression of moral courage, an issue of inner sincerity—manifested in spite of and often in opposition to the ego. (p. 381)

Reik clearly points to the analytic significance of an openness to one's own uniqueness, to one's intuitions. Reik's insights introduce the next attribute of openness to singularity, *solitariness*, the capacity to be alone.

Solitariness: The Capacity to be Alone

Solitariness is an essential but often overlooked characteristic of the facilitating analyst, especially in the current relational ethos that emphasizes the analytic centrality of relatedness, sharing, and intersubjectivity as essential to therapeutic change. Analytic solitariness designates the analyst's capacity to be alone—one's own self—*with* the patient. Solitariness is the ability to hold onto one's own unique perspective; in Reik's terms, this means to listen to one's "own inner voice" while simultaneously listening open-mindedly to the "voice" of another. This is especially true for the coparticipant patient-analyst relationship. Feiner (1979) addresses this crucial dimension of the analyst's therapeutic attitude when he remarks upon the analyst's need to be original:

> The patient does reach us with his presentation of himself, with his necessary "secret lovings and secret hatings." Yet we have secrets of our own as analysts, and one of them is our need to be original. . . . I am referring to our need to be our own persons, our own selves, in connection with the other (the patient) at the same time. (p. 119)

The capacity for solitariness is essential to the experience of solitude, but it is not the same as solitude, for it implies a coparticipant ability to simultaneously listen to another.

For the analyst, solitariness also means the ability to allow and bear without retribution the patient's inevitable psychic assaults, whether they are angry, seductive, dependent, predatory, or passive in character. Further, solitariness implies the ability to feel for the patient's pain and suffering without having to omnipotently or narcissistically take it away— that is, the analyst should *want* to help but not *need* to. Solitariness defines the ability to stand alone and firm in one's analytic convictions, able to confront—in oneself or in one's analytic copartner—whatever requires confrontation regardless of disapproval and the threat of anxiety or psychological pain. Most important, solitariness means having the ability to be alone in the face of the patient's resistance—that is, to be able to steadfastly address resistance without needing to overcome it. Accordingly, solitariness represents one of the most crucial ways for the analyst to facilitate analysis; failure in this area is one of the most frequent reasons why an analysis falters or founders. All too often, as analysts we strive to cure in order to cure our striving rather than that of the patient. All too often, our "need" to cure or to help is in the service of our omnipotence and narcissism rather than our altruism.

For both analyst and patient, solitariness also includes, finally, the ability to accept analytic finitude, the fact that one's work is always unfinished and imperfect. Furthermore, the patient must ultimately leave analysis and the analyst and be on his or her own. The analytic capacity to be alone is closely related to clinical courage, what Grey (1978) refers to as the heroic dimension in psychoanalysis.

Aloneness and relatedness (or separation and connection in Feiner's terms) form an essential psychoanalytic dialectic. In general, if the analyst cannot be alone with the patient, then he or she cannot truly be *with* the patient except in a narcissistic way and thus can not help his or her patients to be alone with themselves either, something patients must learn if they are to claim their own psychic life for themselves.

Fallibility: The Right to be Wrong

Fallibility is closely related to the qualities of psychoanalytic curiosity, solitariness, and clinical innocence and forms an integral aspect of them. Essentially, fallibility implies the right to be wrong; that is, the analyst must be able to entertain multiple perspectives and possibilities, to accept being wrong when he or she errs and to revise his or her interpretations as needed. An attitude of fallibility is suggested in Sullivan's (1954) clinical reminder for analysts to consider if what they hear or observe could possibly have another meaning than the one they see.

Fallibility implies the capacity to allow experience without being concerned about its propriety or reasonableness. To be fallible means to recognize our shared human imperfections, to not have to be right even when the patient transferentially demands it, seductively flatters for it, anxiously cries for it, or angrily threatens to leave the analysis if the analyst does not offer perfection. Fallible analysts accept the inevitable confusion, ambiguity, and messiness of the psychoanalytic process without having to foreclose them with definitive interpretations. In other words, analysts must accept that there will always be some ineluctable, unfathomable mystery about the other, that we can never exhaust our study of his or her complexity and unique individuality; and the recognition that, in the final analysis, that there will always be something ineffable about the coparticipant process of psychoanalytically coming to know another.

As with the other aspects of openness to singularity, as the analyst develops the analytic freedom and his or her ability to be fallible, these capacities are also fostered in the patient, who always suffers problems with the reality of uncertainty. Patients, whatever other difficulties they may have, invariably have problems with their fallibility. All patients suffer to some extent from narcissism, grandiosity, or strivings for perfection. This is why it is so critical for the analyst to develop a working acceptance of his or her own imperfection and fallibility.

Spontaneity

By *spontaneity* I mean unpremeditated responsiveness to the moment, a readiness to accept and follow through on one's immediate experience. Of course, being spontaneous is not the same as being impulsive or neglecting one's analytic responsibilities. Instead, spontaneity openly and freely flows from the personal self, from what Wolstein (1985, 1987) calls the analyst's psychic center. It is different from what compulsively erupts from countertransference or counterresistance, from the psychic dimension of the interpersonal self.

As Wolstein (1977b) points out,

> Spontaneity is not . . . a wild animal that needs to be trapped, tran-
> quilized, caged. . . . It arises, rather, as a generic trait of the human
> psyche, it is directly acquired through natural endowment. It char-
> acterizes the immediate subject of original, psychic process—
> unique, individual, active. . . . And so, spontaneity does not appear
> in the psychoanalyst or in his patient as a matter of caprice, whim,
> fashion, indulgence. It represents a genuine aspect of the human psy-
> che, to be deflected and deformed only at the risk of either or both
> coparticipants crippling their serious efforts at psychoanalytic
> inquiry. (p. 408)

These words were Wolstein's response to Sullivan's advocacy of a prescriptive and manipulative technique, as embodied in his clinical apho-
rism that everything is spontaneous yet nothing is spontaneous. Wolstein
points to the therapeutic benefits of a direct human-natural psychoanalytic approach to treatment. Spontaneity, in fact, forms an integral aspect
of openness to singularity, essential to the facilitation of analytic aliveness.

Feiner's (1979) concept of the "anxiety of influence" addresses an
aspect of the analyst's difficulties in this area. Feiner discusses how the
analyst's fear of influencing the patient may countertransferentially curb
his or her creative responsivity and provoke, as Tauber (1979) points out,
a false view of this creative responsivity as itself being neurotic countertransference.

However, spontaneity always involves the personally unique becoming
the interpersonally unique; it implies a willingness to be personally
revealed, to open one's singularity to the analytic scrutiny and potential
disapproval of his or her coparticipant partner. Spontaneous relatedness
is thus authentic relatedness. Induplicable and unique to a given interpersonal moment or juncture, analytic spontaneity always conveys freshness
and tends to carry surprise, for the other as well as for its originator.

Moments of analytic spontaneity may be hard to capture in words, but
they are often the most alive ones in an analysis. They are often difficult,
if not impossible, to recapture. They are lived, undergone, and then gone
(although leaving resultant change in both coparticipants). Words are
inevitably incommensurate to the elusive essence of these experiences.
Following such experiences, we are often left with a certainty of analytic
occurrence, of analytic life being lived fully; but of being unable to know
or communicate it syntaxically, or only able to approximate it in terms
that are inevitably pale or inadequate. Yet these experiences are no less
valuable and therapeutic because they cannot be captured precisely in
words.

OPENNESS TO SINGULARITY AND CLINICAL INQUIRY

The five interrelated capacities that constitute *openness to singularity* emphasize the specific, singular, or individual in the analytic experience. Openness to the singularity of both the analyst's and the patient's uniqueness and to the uniqueness of their interaction at any given moment characterizes the coparticipatory relatedness of a given psychoanalytic dyad. And it includes the unique interpersonal history of the coparticipants— their unique history of past interpersonal relations. Though the constituent elements of openness to singularity may be considered individually, they represent aspects of one another and form an integral whole.

Obviously, therapeutic growth and self-transformation depend upon many factors, not just openness to singularity. They are always poised on a dialectic of openness to singularity (unique individuality) and openness to similarity (consensual adaptability), of openness to the improvisatory and to the methodical. When an analysis is stuck or derailed, one of the problems is usually an inhibition or compromise of openness to singularity. For example, an analysis may become an unfocused inquiry without therapeutic effects, or it may become a "stereotyped" inquiry which the analyst insists on forcing the patient into a prescribed diagnosis, metapsychology, or methodology. Another example is that therapeutic situation where there is a ritual avoidance of central dynamic issues by analyst or patient (or both). "Stereotyped" analyses also include such clinical situations as the "bogged-down" or stalemated analysis; the all-too-common "constricted" analysis, with its overly conventional focus, narrow scope, and avoidant tone; the "flat" analysis, which, as its name implies, is depressive or dispirited in content and function; and the "endless" analysis, with its two subtypes, the "hateful integration," in which patient and analyst are trapped in an interlocking sado-masochistic relationship, and the "lovey-dovey," or mutually idealizing, experience.

Whatever other difficulties these and similar situations represent, they generally reflect pathologies of openness to singularity—blockages of the analytic search for the individual and singular. In two clinical papers, Cooper and Witenberg (1983, 1985) cogently detail the facilitating effects of imaginatively reconstructing or visualizing patient's narrative accounts and of forming an overall picture of the person in his or her specific and singular modes of relating to others. They explain how failures in these processes lead to "bogged-down" treatments. A cornerstone of their recommendations is the focus on the specifics, or interpersonally unique experiences, of patients' therapeutic adaptations. The formation of a therapeutic overview and the stimulation of the analyst's therapeutic curiosity involve an interest in and attention to the patient's individual circumstances and experiences. Without an interest in the singularity of the person and his or her unique experiences, inquiry will ossify.

Constriction or inhibition of openness to singularity derives from: (1) warped or inhibited development of one or more of its component abilities in the analyst or patient; (2) the dynamic intrusion of resistance, counterresistance, countertransference, anxiety, and apprehension; and (3) the negative impact of restrictive psychoanalytic paradigms or models of inquiry.

The personal development of openness to singularity is most centrally addressed in one's self-analysis or personal analysis and also in one's training and supervisory experiences. Cooper and Witenberg, addressing the issue of curiosity and its stimulation, point out ways in which supervision can quicken the development of this attitude. They limit their efforts to the specific application of curiosity to extratransference narratives. However, similar supervisory attention can be directed to the development of an openness to singularity in transference (and countertransference) experience and in the unique personal and interpersonal aspects of the patient.

Counterresistance and countertransference interference with openness to singularity requires the same self-monitoring that other aspects of counterresistance or countertransference call for, an openness to openness to singularity, as it were. Analysts need to examine their ability to function in an open manner, and if they find themselves incapable of such openness, they should question, even in coinquiry with their patients, why this is. Analysts may fail to achieve such openness or inquire into the reasons for such failure, not because they want to avoid knowing others, but because they wish to avoid knowing themselves. We can only truly know another to the extent we allow ourselves to see ourselves in them and to know ourselves in response to them.

Fear of openness to singularity finds its source not simply in the anxiety of bad or forbidden experience but also in the apprehension of new experience. As discussed in chapter 4, analysts and patients fear unformed, unfamiliar experience as well as repressed experience. Schachtel refers to this fear of the unpredictable and unfamiliar as embeddedness anxiety, and Fromm refers to it as the fear of freedom. As Schachtel (1959) points out, "Man is afraid that without the support of his accustomed attitudes, perspective, and labels he will fall into an abyss or flounder in the pathless" (p. 195). As he defined it, "The unknown danger . . . is the new, unknown state of being when leaving a particular constellation of embeddedness" (p. 47).

The processes comprising openness to singularity represent personal qualities that are not the exclusive property of analysts of any particular psychoanalytic orientation. Nevertheless, some models of analytic inquiry may inhibit, circumscribe, or constrain the expression of these capacities while other models may facilitate their emergence and development.

A detailed comparative analysis of how the technical precepts of the different schools of psychoanalysis impact on openness to singularity would be fruitful but goes beyond the exploratory scope of this book. Here, I will very briefly view openness to singularity from the broad perspectives of the three inclusive models of psychoanalytic praxis outlined in earlier chapters (see especially chapter 3): (1) the nonparticipant mirror, (2) participant-observation, and (3) coparticipation.

How do these models discourage or encourage openness to singularity in the analytic experience? The *nonparticipant-mirror* model, in its focus on regressive process, free associational technique, and an analytic attitude of evenly hovering attention, fosters an analytic openness to singularity while also emphasizing -analytic reserve and restraint, and the authority, anonymity, and neutrality of the analyst. The *participant-observer* model also simultaneously facilitates and inhibits analytic openness to singularity. Sullivan's focus on clarity of communication and his notion of an active and detailed inquiry promote an openness to singularity. Yet Sullivan's notion of the analyst as expert and his explicit repudiation of unique individuality as an analytic parameter limit openness to singularity. Similarly, the implicitly authoritarian praxis of many object-relationists inhibits openness to singularity, as does the contemporary interpersonalist tendency to reduce the self and individual experience to the push and pull of the interpersonal field.

The *coparticipant model* of praxis facilitates analytic openness to singularity, both personal and interpersonal, as evidenced in Ferenczi's emphasis on mutuality in analysis. Wolstein's concepts of unique individuality and psychic realism, and Levenson's perspectivism, transactional realism, and pursuit of the analytic particular, also point in the same direction, as does the work of many other coparticipant analysts. All emphasize individual uniqueness, personal responsibility and responsiveness, creative self-expression, and personal freedom of praxis and belief.

Openness to singularity is obviously not a matter of technical precept, but of personal attribute and attitude. In pointing to its importance as a crucial aspect of analytic facilitation, I want to emphasize the central importance in therapeutic growth and analytic aliveness of the personal self and the real relationship: the fundamental reality and analytic centrality of personal individuality.

CHAPTER 11

Therapeutic Processes in the Analytic Working Space

ANXIETY AND THE ANALYTIC WORK SPACE

The conscious and unconscious analytic space between terror and despair defines the range of effective analytic work. It is within this *analytic working space,* bounded by too much and too little anxiety, that patients and analysts are able to live and work through their respective neuroses and narcissisms. When there is too much analytic anxiety, whether on the side of the patient or the analyst, effective coinquiry disintegrates or is shifted into resistance or counterresistance. That is, either one or both coparticipants become preoccupied with restoring self-esteem and avoiding any more anxiety and loss of self-esteem. Analytic communication and learning is handicapped or halted until one coparticipant is able to help the other reduce his or her anxiety and regain his or her sense of self-esteem. More often than not this is the role of the analyst, but the patient may also be cast in this role when he or she is temporarily the more mature of the two. When there is too little anxiety, for either patient or analyst, the interpersonal self and its defensive operations hold sway, and the patient's or analyst's neurosis and narcissism remain unchallenged and unanalyzed—patient and analyst collude self-protectively, and analytic communication and learning is minimal or illusory.

Harry Stack Sullivan, the psychoanalytic theorist who most extensively studied and developed perhaps the most comprehensive understanding of clinical anxiety, considered it the chief culprit in human psychological difficulty and suffering. Sullivan stressed the importance of attending to the ebb and flow of anxious experience in the therapeutic setting. Intimately linked to the processes constituting self-esteem, anxiety is a major disjunctive or disruptive psychological force, in life and in analysis. Comprising a number of dysphoric and terrifying feeling states, including horror, terror, loathing, shame, and extreme fear verging on panic, sudden or severe anxiety can approach nightmarish proportions. (For a fuller and more detailed account of Sullivan's theory of anxiety and its implications for coparticipant inquiry, see chapter 4.)

Patients and analysts vary in the breadth of their analytic working space—in their potential for coinquiry. Some are remarkably open to analytic anxiety and able to tolerate it well; others can bear only very little and almost instantly seek emotional comfort, or fearful withdrawal. For each analytic dyad, then, the interpersonal selves, or security needs, of analyst and patient codetermine or circumscribe a dyadic working space, unique to them and defined by the intersecting security needs (or resistances and counterresistances) of the two coparticipants. This constitutes the particular *coparticipant working space* within which each particular dyad works.

For each analytic dyad, throughout the course of an analysis, the work of inquiry tends to move in unpredictable pattern from one pole of this coparticipantly created *analytic working space* to the other—from terror, or too much anxiety, to despair and dread, or not enough anxiety. Of course, there is always the analytic mandate to work nearer the pole of terror—to work at the edge of conscious experience and thus, at times, to experience the terror or anxiety of dissociated (repressed) or selectively ignored experience. There is also the analyst's mandate to widen or expand the analytic working space; in other words, the analyst should work toward developing greater tolerance of psychoanalytic growth and its concomitant anxiety and psychic pain.

A crucial aspect of an analyst's therapeutic skill is his or her ability to steer an analytic course between the extremes of too much anxiety (terror) and too little. Crucial also is the analyst's ability to foster the development of this skill in the patient. Not infrequently, this process works in inverse order; that is, the coparticipant patient encourages or otherwise attempts to foster the coparticipant analyst's personal and interpersonal growth, including his or her ability to better tolerate the fears or terrors of analytic change—of venturing into unknown or forbidden new ground or territory.

Neurotic patients, particularly self-centered narcissists, highly sensitive and deeply private schizoid individuals, critical help-rejecting depressives, and controlling obsessives typically have a very narrow analytic working space. They can take very little anxiety; given their grandiose and irrational sense of themselves, it takes very little to make them anxious. In Sullivan's (1953) terms, these patients may be said to have a very steep anxiety gradient, and analytic work with them is focused on securing their trust, and making and maintaining empathic contact with a profoundly injured, vulnerable, and defensive interpersonal self. In other words, analysis with these patients requires very patient, sensitive work and constant and careful attention to subtle issues of self-esteem, often over a long period of time.

EMPATHY AND ENGAGEMENT

The more severely neurotic or narcissistic patients are, the more insecure and fragile their subjective sense of self-worth, the less they are able to tolerate confrontation or questioning of their subjective perspective or their defensive ways of relating. These defensive ways are often expressed in highly demanding, arrogant, or grandiose and angry ways as well as in more subtly exploitative ways, in what Sullivan (1953) called preying on sympathy. Such patients find it difficult to tolerate interpretive interventions or relational interactions that confront them with their forbidden and dissociated infantile grandiosity or their repressed developmental needs for love and acceptance.   Needless to say, this places severe limitations on the work. Analytic efforts, particularly in the beginning of treatment, are often focused on the vicissitudes of the interpersonal self, rather than on those of the personal or relational selves.

The analyst's task of navigating between too much anxiety and too little becomes then very difficult and requires centered selfness and robust self-esteem in the analyst if the coparticipant inquiry is to be successful. This is not to say that patients cannot be engaged or confronted; in fact, I suggest that a therapy emphasizing a highly personal engagement of the patient is the most effective.

Such engagement requires, however, that the analyst be highly flexible, capable of moving rapidly and sensitively from one pole of the coparticipant working space to the other. Therapeutic engagement also demands that the analyst be alert and attentive to often subtle shifts in the patient's self-esteem. Above all, it requires that the analyst possess the solidity of self-esteem, personal centeredness, and relative freedom from narcissism to autonomously and authentically stand firm in his or her clinical intuitions and convictions, while remaining open to the patient's singularity and subjectivity. The analyst must confront the often disturbing transference resistances of patients. It is precisely this threat that recommends to many the safer, but less alive analytic technique typical of nonparticipant inquiry. Though less comfortable or comforting, a more active and challenging approach to patients, in my view, makes for optimal analytic progress.

However, when the analyst's interventions or interactive invitations (questioning, interpreting, or ways of relating, etc.) create too much anxiety (whatever its roots), the analyst must resume empathic connectedness with his or her patient's interpersonal self and subjective perspective. That is, the analyst must restore the patient's sense of security and self-esteem, often by relating to the patient's defensive need to have the analyst see things from his or her self-centered perspective and to acknowledge the analyst's "failure" to do so. All this fosters the patient's ability: (a) to continue the coparticipant analytic work, to engage in self-inquiry, free association, interpretive formulation, and in shared inquiry into his or her copartner's (i.e., the analyst's) psychology; and (b) to remain open to the analyst's interpretations and therapeutic interactions and to his or her own intuitive understandings. In short, the analytic work space is widened, and the patient is helped to work ever closer to the edge of terror.

Although it is therapeutically crucial to empathically feel one's way into the patient's subjective (defensive) perspective, one must also confront its difficulties and distortions. It is incumbent on the analyst to facilitate a widening of the patient's often narrow perspective and to help the patient develop a more complete and complex understanding of the world and how it works (including the psychology of his or her analyst). The patient's point of view (like that of the analyst) is often distorted, incomplete, and solipsistic.

Coparticipant inquiry is a complex analytic dance that moves back and forth in often unpredictable and always unique ways from one end of the analytic work space to the other. The analyst must be able to see things from the perspective of his or her patient, yet it is equally important for the analyst to be unafraid to assert his or her own perspective. Otherwise treatment devolves into a solipsistic exercise and disregards the patient's need to grow and to shed his or her childhood egocentricity. Both the analyst's inability to see the patient's point of view and *only* seeing things from the patient's point of view represent the analyst's countertransferential coparticipation, which requires analytic attention and exploration.

It is essential for the analyst to remain experientially close to the patient's anxiety and apprehension—to be attentive to the subtle movements of the patient's anxiety—in order for the patient to be able to tolerate the rigors of analytic work. Neurotic personalities have fragile self-esteem; working with them requires considerable attention and empathy with their seemingly self-assured and "normal" yet basically vulnerable interpersonal selves. Working with narcissistic individuals, for example, requires considerable support of their narcissistic defenses. When a therapeutic intervention has subjectively been too hurtful or stressful for the patient, as revealed in his or her verbal reports, transference enactments, symbolic symptomatology, or dream life, there is a therapeutic need to shift attention to an empathic restoration of an approving relationship.

When the analyst's interpretation of a patient's defensive dynamic leads to further reactive and defensive symptomatology on the part of the patient, the analyst can then interpret the patient's wish or need for empathic relatedness. This strengthens the preexisting empathic connection between patient and analyst and implicitly meets early archaic needs for empathic resonance. The analyst's ability to be open and nondefensive about the patient's anxiety and defensive self-protective behavior, to see the patient's point of view, and to stay within the analytic work space is what allows the patient to eventually internalize that original interpretation because the patient now feels understood. This process eventually leads to a gradual release of defensiveness, for the patient gradually begins to realize that he or she is acceptable without his or her defenses.

On this point, Sullivan (*1940*) observed that

> until a patient has seen clearly and unmistakenly a concrete example of the way in which unresolved situations from the distant past color the perception of present situations and overcomplicates action in them, there can be no material reorganization of personality, no therapeutically satisfactory expansion of the self, no significant insight into the complexities of one's performances or into the unexpected and often disconcerting behavior of others concerned. Up to this point, there is nothing significantly unique in the treatment situation; afterward, however, the integration with [the analyst] becomes a situation of unprecedented freedom from restraints on the manifestation of constructive impulses. This is the indirect result of the changes in the self system. The patient has finally learnt that more security may ensue form abandoning a complex security-seeking process than was ever achieved by it. This information is in itself an addition to security and a warrant for confronting other anxiety-provoking situations to discover the factors in them which are being experienced as a threat. [The analyst's] reiterated statement as to the way by which one gains mental health now takes on something of the meaning which he has striven to communicate. The patient is beginning to understand what is sought, and its virtue. Up to now, the patient has been literally in Groddeck's words "lived by unknown and uncontrollable forces," however elaborately this fact was concealed from awareness. (pp. *205–206*)

Interpretations and interactive invitations the patient initially sees as insensitive or unempathic may gradually be accepted if the analyst is emotionally aware of the empathic rupture and conveys his or her nondefensive, centered understanding of the patient's defensive need. When people feel respected and cared about, which for many patients may take a very long time, they can accept new information about themselves even when it hurts.

RESISTANCE AND RESPONSIBILITY

It is important to distinguish between hurting a person in the sense of hurting their feelings, and doing harm or injury to that person. Hurting a patient's feelings, though painful, is often an unavoidable aspect of analytic work. This hurtfulness is different from harming the patient in some significant aspect of their life—of relating to one's patients in a manner that is inimical to their best interests. In the latter case, the harm done to the patient goes beyond the discomfort of hurt feelings.

The readiness with which many people blame others for their hurt feelings reflects the other-directed and outer-directed nature of our culture. We can see this even in our language; for example, we say we have been "made" anxious by someone as though we did not ultimately generate our anxiety ourselves.

Frequently, patients' complaints, anger, or "disappointment" with the analyst represent defensive efforts to force the analyst to treat them in less confronting ways. The patient, in essence, attempts to gain a sense of self-esteem through manipulation of the interpersonal environment. The patient externalizes his or her problems; anxiety thus becomes the fault of others' insensitivity or hostility, not the failure of one's own security, an unhappy consequence of one's low self-esteem. In this way, the patient attempts to secure self-esteem without having to examine the personal roots of his or her anxiety. Instead of exploring the inner sources of their anxiety, patients focus on getting their environment (i.e., the analyst) to change. Interpretations along these lines aim to strengthen the autonomous personal self rather than reassuring the insecure interpersonal self.

Coparticipantly working through our anxieties and defenses is frightening, and manipulating or coercing others into taking responsibility for our experience may seem easier. However, it keeps us insecure and dependent and fails to achieve the intended goal.

Patients often are hampered in both their interpersonal responsiveness and their personal sense of responsibility; in fact, deficiencies in responsivity and responsibility are characteristic symptoms of their pathology. Optimally, the analyst (who invariably has his or her own problems with these dimensions of human experience) is able to foster the patient's growth in both aspects of this analytic dialectic. The patient can then develop a greater capacity to be responsive to his or her interpersonal world and become more open to the influence of others while also being aware of his or her own experience and personal capacities.

Historically, impersonal psychoanalytic notions of the analytic work space resulted in an eclipse of the other in the analytic situation. With the development of interpersonal and relational concepts of psychoanalytic inquiry, however, there has been a tendency to focus one-sidedly on the other's impact on the self. This has resulted in a psychoanalytic eclipse of the personal self and an exaggerated concern with the interpersonal self. In a sense, this mirrors the tendency of patients to externalize their problems, to locate their neurosis in the interpersonal influence of their significant others. In contrast, coparticipant inquiry recognizes the analytic importance of concepts of personal responsibility and of the personal sources of both psychic difficulty and psychic strength.

With certain severely narcissistic patients, including those of a predominately obsessional or depressive character, analysis may require protracted, very long periods of simply siding with their narcissistic defenses because these patients often cannot bear to have their defenses or the underlying forbidden childhood needs interpreted or in any way noted. The more fragile a patient's self-esteem, the slower and gentler the process of confronting the patient with his or her narcissistic defenses and underlying archaic narcissism must be. Some patients exhibit an almost impossible analytic working space—the band of acceptable intervention is too narrow to allow any therapeutic leverage. Often, the analyst's unconscious and uncomfortable appraisal of this fact causes fear and countertransference restriction or countertransferential overactivity, all of which can move the analyst to cross the boundaries of the analytic working space and to precipitate a temporary or protracted analytic impasse or transference-countertransference interlock (Wolstein *1959*) and even, in some instances, termination of the analysis.

COPARTICIPANT INQUIRY AND COUNTERTRANSFERENCE

The analyst's anxiety and defensiveness, as it emerges in the countertransference and counterresistance, may further restrict patients' already narrow analytic working space. The neuroses of patient and analyst may, in fact, intersect in such ways that they preclude the possibility of successful work together. Their coparticipant analytic working space may be too narrow for effective work. The analysis becomes mired in the collusive defensive play of mutually comforting security operations. If such a situation becomes chronic, the patient may seek a different analytic situation; one or both of the coparticipants experience their dyadic fit as incompatible. However, the analyst's or patient's analysis of the transference and countertransference may widen the coinquiry sufficiently to begin or to resume productive and effective analytic work.

The repressed forbidden feelings and desires of patients often evoke similar or reciprocal countertransferential anxieties in the analyst, along with his or her unique pattern of defenses. In addition, patients' defensive narcissism—their contempt, coerciveness, and arrogance—often psychically wound the insecure analyst and provoke anxiety.

It can be emotionally trying for the analyst to be treated relentlessly as stupid, inferior, or inept. Analysts often sense that they run the risk of incurring rejection, contempt, or ridicule if they express or reveal their human fallibility and vulnerability. Analysts anticipate hurt pride and lowered self-esteem if they were to disclose their own forbidden childhood wants or their personal imperfections and limitations. These analytic anxieties may, in turn, provoke the analyst's retaliatory rage, detachment, or emotional withdrawal and thus lead to rejection of the patient. The submissive and masochistic analyst may deal with patients' hostility and contempt by attempting to appease the patient and ingratiate himself or herself. Some analysts meet patients' hostility with an effort to identify with their aggressor and to vicariously live out their own dissociated childhood wishes and wants. These and similar countertransference attitudes interfere with the analyst's empathy with his or her patient's anxieties. Unless worked through, they will block the analyst's ability to engage in a fruitful coinquiry with his or her patient.

A frequent theme in analysis is that of control or power. It is important for the analyst to avoid or to work through being controlled (i.e., intimidated or coerced) or needing to exert power over the patient. This dynamic is often overlooked, with resultant impoverishment of the analytic possibilities of the coparticipant inquiry. Though the problem of power is not unique to the treatment of neurotic conditions, it is exaggerated in working with obsessional, depressive, and narcissistic patients. The grandiose analyst is often provoked into countertransference acting-out when he or she neurotically needs to *overcome* the patient's analytic recalcitrance and stubborn resistance. Analysts must realize that treatment is a matter of the patient needing to change, not the analyst needing the patient to change. This also holds true for the coparticipant patient. The analyst may need to change, but the patient's experienced need for the analyst to change in order to avoid his or her own anxiety (or responsibility for it) represents a coercive externalization of the patient's psychopathology and is obviously a transference issue that calls for coparticipant analytic exploration.

Unresolved omnipotent strivings in the analyst are fertile ground for countertransference provocation by such patients, given their self-centeredness, controlling grandiosity, and often impossible demands. The analyst's power needs and narcissism may lead him or her to an analytic authoritarianism, whether *sadistic*—manifested in angry humiliating, blaming, or rejecting the patient—or *masochistic*—evident in appeasing or ingratiating behaviors, infantilizing the patient, analytic timidity, and in feelings of guilt, inferiority, and ineptitude.

If the analyst and the patient fail to attend to countertransference and counterresistance factors, this will further restrict the already narrow coparticipant working space characteristic of many narcissistic, obsessional, or depressive patients. Thus the analyst must observe and work through his or her neurotic countertransference and counterresistance. And in this process, the analyst may coparticipantly invite the patient's coanalysis of his or her countertransference.

Although countertransference analysis plays a critical role in the treatment of many depressive, narcissistic, and obsessional patients, because of their separation anxiety and their anxiety about imperfections in themselves or others, these patients tend to resist countertransference or counterresistance analysis as well as transference analysis. When the analyst's neurotic needs dovetail with the patient's reluctance to inquire into countertransference, then the analyst countertransferentially reinforces this disinclination. Moreover, analysts, like patients, may be loath to inquire into their *own* resistance to countertransference analysis and into the patient's similar resistance.

However, analysts who are open to coparticipant inquiry into countertransference experience provide the patient with a therapeutic model of healthy functioning, and the possibility of being inner-directed and self-expressive. Of course, if the patient becomes too anxious about such an inquiry and narrows the coparticipant work space, the analyst must back off, stop confronting the patient with his or her psychopathology or disclosing his or her own, and temporarily meet the patient's current defensive need. Nevertheless, in my experience, all patients, even the most severely narcissistic or schizoid, can tolerate some coparticipant analytic inquiry, even if initially only to a limited degree.

The analyst's anxieties and countertransference may express themselves in analytic actions that are too confronting and generate too much analytic anxiety. The insecure and grandiose analyst may countertransferentially respond to his or her patient's irrational dependency and sense of entitlement by reactively becoming hard-nosed and tough. The analyst may then exhort the patient to just grow up. This is good advice, but it is never taken. After all, merely willing to grow up is not enough; one has to live it in order to make it one's own. Counterresistance may also be expressed in therapeutic passivity or in an approach that is too comforting. The analyst may defensively deal with his or her inability to accept his or her imperfections by denying their existence and by insisting on being the benign or sensitive empathic analyst who can fulfill what are actually impossible demands.

Analysts' empathy for their patients may be beneficially rooted in a genuine compassion for the patients. But empathy can also be premised on a defensive dynamic. The seeming sensitivity of the empathic analyst may actually be countertransferential in origin. For example, it can represent an anxious collusion with a patient's defensive demand for endless empathy to avoid confronting his or her problems. The analyst may also be living out his or her wish to be therapeutically needed and then presents an image of himself or herself as sensitive and thoughtful. As a result, the analyst can vicariously enjoy the sense of security afforded the patient (to give the patient what he or she wants to be given), and deny his or her own unconscious hostility and actual hatred of others. Of course, patients need the genuine (nondefensive) sensitivity of a caring and empathic therapist. What is said here of the analyst applies equally to the patient, something often overlooked by analysts who do not work in a coparticipant way. However, whether analysts (or patients) are aware of them or not, coparticipant processes continue to flow in both analytic directions.

Though active engagement with the patient is essential and judicious confrontation of the patient's defenses facilitates analytic progress, the analyst must remain aware of the excessive and disjunctive use of such confrontation. The most important therapeutic lesson of theorists of the self, such as Carl Rogers, lies in their insistence on being sensitive to the therapeutic interplay of primitive aspects of the interpersonal self and on carefully monitoring the anxiety surrounding dissociated yearnings and needs. To approach patients in a manner that ignores or minimizes their vulnerable self-esteem and expects more of them than they can psychically tolerate is to fall prey to the *fallacy of adultilization*. This invariably results in a neurotic replay of early shaming experience, further repressing the patient's infantile grandiosity; it also further strengthens the patient's defense structure.

Too bold an inquiry into patients' defenses invariably strengthens their hold upon the patient. Analyses that are rigidly aggressive—too confronting, generating too much analytic anxiety, lead to a disjunctive or disintegrative analytic situation. The coparticipant work space becomes too narrow to be workable: the patient takes refuge in new and more complex resistances, stalls the work, engages in power struggles, or in other ways blocks productive analytic work; alternatively, the patient simply leaves the field and quits.

On the other hand, therapeutic preoccupation with the interpersonal self and an overly supportive approach that calls for unabated empathy with the patient's subjective experience runs the risk of reinforcing childhood experiences. In this case, the analyst overlooks the patient's developmental need to grow beyond his or her childhood fixations.

The analyst's empathy with the patient's interpersonal self must be balanced by an understanding of the patient's sensual, relational, and personal selves, the developmental strivings toward physical satisfaction, relational intimacy, and personal fulfillment (cf. Fiscalini *1991*). The analyst's empathy must extend beyond the patient's security needs and also include the patient's needs for an expanded and enriched living. To focus empathy exclusively on the patient's interpersonal self essentially dismisses the patient's psychic resources and potentials—his or her personal self. The analyst in that case may be said to fall into *the fallacy of infantilization*.

When the analyst becomes too concerned with the patient's analytic anxieties, he or she abandons the patient's repressed needs for psychological growth and courts the development of analytic despair. The analytic work space remains fixated near the pole of despair, with its sense of analytic work undone, of life unlived (though this may be outside the patient's awareness). Patients who need and want more will leave the analysis. Less assertive patients may lapse into a comforting and protracted codependency. In these and similar cases, the patient and analyst may consider the treatment a viable one, but personal growth is nonexistent or illusory.

The working through of analytic impasses, and the analyst's countertransference adultilizing and infantilizing misjudgments, emphasizes the importance of the analyst's sensitive monitoring of the coparticipant work space, of the play between too much and too little analytic anxiety. Much of the therapeutic skill in working with peoples' problems in living lies in the analyst's ability to attend to patients' therapeutic need to get in touch with their early repressed desires and beliefs and their need to grow and develop beyond them. This clinical dialectic is mirrored in the crucial dialectic of comforting and confronting patients. In other words, the coparticipant inquiry must take into equal account the analytic vicissitudes of the personal and the interpersonal selves of patient and analyst.

THE ANALYSIS OF RESISTANCE

Just as patients need to reclaim their early narcissism, they also need to transform it into more mature forms of relating to others. This is not a matter of subjugating one's individuality, of adapting to society's or the analyst's standards. Rather it is a developmental need to unfold one's individuality. It is as important for the analyst to empathize with patients' dissociated developmental needs for limits as it is for him or her to empathize with patients' need for unconditional acceptance. The analyst should assist the patient in implementing his or her maturing abilities to love, to feel, and to embrace a world of many perspectives, not just the one he or she is most familiar with. To do otherwise is to condemn the patient to a solipsistic life. The goal of realistic maturity and acceptance of human imperfection is best accomplished by an active and at times confronting engagement of the patient, including the confrontation and interpretation of the patient's defensive structure.

It might be argued that my recommendations for active interpretation of the harmfulness of patients' defenses and of the patient's developmental need to relinquish infantile forms of need satisfaction are countertherapeutic and reflect a maturity morality; that this approach is countertransferentially motivated. However, in my view the *failure* to interpret patients' defensiveness and need to outgrow their early childhood yearnings is countertransferential. Analysts do not have to maintain empathy with the patient's immature perspective, which could re-create the same problem that led to the development of substitutive defensiveness in the first place. In other words, it could keep the patient from developing appropriate competencies and accepting actual imperfections and limitations. Ultimately, this approach ignores the patient's psychic resources, thus reinforcing the patient's neurotic formulation that he or she can only cope with life on a defensive basis.

The patient's defenses will not, as some believe, wither away once the patient or analyst gets in touch with his or her dissociated early needs. These defenses must be identified and interpreted in all their self-protective and substitutive function, their self-defeating nature, and their harmful impact on others.

Security operations or defenses are self-perpetuating and may even become functionally autonomous. They form an integral part of patients' interpersonal "warp and woof" and they do not simply disappear through empathic inattention. The patient must come to understand and to live through with some pain the patterned intrapsychic and interpsychic features of his or her defensive structure, laying bare their psychological necessity, meaning, dynamics, and effects.

Of course, defense or resistance analysis always proceeds within the context of the analysis of transference need, of the dissociated and not fully lived, anxious needs hidden within the patient's defensive self-system. To focus on the analysis of defensive behavior and experience without the concomitant analysis of its anxious underpinnings produces too much anxiety and ultimately is demoralizing or discouraging. Conversely, to focus on the patient's anxiety and transference need without concomitant attention to the problematics of his or her defensiveness leads to analytic despair; the patient feels that he or she is falsely accepted and not really known.

Patients work through their defenses in the living through process and in interpretive analysis. Defensive or security operations cannot be overcome whether by attempts at cajolery, coercion, moralistic blaming, bribery, or "appeal to reason." Such tactics reflect the analyst's anxiety and countertransferential wish to deflect or get rid of these defenses rather than to analyze their meaning or function in the patient's psychic life. And such attempts will simply, as Sullivan (1953) warns us, promote the development of even more complex, recondite, and entrenched defenses—of an even more complicated set or series of defensive operations.

The effective analysis of defenses will, as Sullivan's (1953) Theorem of Escape predicts, invariably provoke anxiety, apprehension (cf. Fiscalini 1991), and further defensive symptomatology. These are substitute escapes into a spiraling set of secondary defensive cognitions, feelings, and behaviors (and their rationalizations). These secondary defenses (i.e., defenses of defenses) and their anxious underpinnings must also be worked through and lived through. Patients' reactive symptomatology must not be mistaken for a response to the analyst's failure to empathize with the patient's infantile needs. Instead, this symptomatology reflects secondary anxiety—a threat to the defensive structure, not the primary threat of obliterative disapproval of early needs.

It is essential for analysts to engage their coparticipant partners in a mutual exploration of the myriad facets of the patient's defenses—constantly moving forward and creating anxiety, then pulling back and reducing anxiety, then forward again, and so forth. The clinical specifics of the coinquiry into patients' defensive structures and residual childhood needs—its spirit, timing, procedural patterning, sequence of therapeutic processes, and method and manner of exploration—cannot be predetermined or in any way prescribed. When therapeutic, it emerges organically from the spontaneous thrust of the coparticipant inquiry.

In coparticipant inquiry in the analytic work space, the analyst's clinical decisions and actions develop intuitively from the analyst's individual analytic sensibility and clinical sensitivity. Rather than follow a prescribed technique, coparticipant analysts (or more accurately, analysts working in a coparticipant way), rely on their own singular qualities of mind and heart. These analysts rely on their uniquely individual clinical intuition, imagination, judgment, and experience in deciding issues such as how hard to press the patient at a given point or on a given issue or how venturesome to be; how to assess or estimate the patient's (or one's own) ability to tolerate anxiety and the disorganization of analytic growth; how much to question, and what to ask; how much to explore an emergent analytic theme, and whether to defer exploration to another time.

Much of what is effective in analytic treatment stems from the analyst's ability to be free of countertransferential or counterresistant aggravation of the patient's neurotic resistances. For example, if a patient becomes angry, derogatory, or condescending because an aspect of his or her protective defensive wall has been breached, the analyst needs to accept this nondefensively, inquire into its genesis and function, consider its countertransference or transference-countertransference aspects, analyze them, move to heal the patient's self-esteem injury, and acknowledge the empathic rupture if this is therapeutically necessary, moving back and forth between the boundaries of the coparticipant work space, between terror and despair, striving always to move from the dread of unfulfillment toward the terror of personal growth.

Regardless of their specific pattern, all psychoanalyses involve the patient's need to work through his or her self-defeating, maladaptive patterns of living and to live through and resolve his or her archaic anxieties in order to live out developmentally stunted needs and allow new ones to emerge.

The analysis of neurotic patients requires, among other things, a flexible and open dialectical attention to defensive and infantile narcissism, to developmental needs for limits and for boundless cherishing, to spoiling and to shaming experience, to the patient's subjective perspective and to those of the analyst's alternatives, and to despair and terror as they define the coparticipant working space. And in the work that takes place in this space, it is important for the analyst not to lose sight of the interpersonal self's reciprocal needs for limitless acceptance and for acceptable limits.

Often patients will talk about wanting to be accepted "as they are" by others in their life and by the analyst. This may represent *defensive desire* or *true desire*. The former refers to the patient's defensive wish to avoid anxiety—to be accepted "as is," defenses and all. Now, this is impossible, for the patient's defenses are often self-destructive and destructive to others. Thus, to love or accept the defenses is to abandon the patient's human potentials. The analyst can, however, accept and love the patient's *need* for such defenses—his or her need, however neurotic or narcissistic, to protect himself or herself (or, more accurately, to protect his or her self-image). It is seldom the painful truth of an interpretation or analytic interaction that proves so intolerable or difficult to internalize. Rather it is the surrounding countertransference feelings—the anger, envy, fear, irritation, contempt, judgmentalness, etc.—that are so often an integral, but disclaimed, part of analytic interventions.

Countertransference analysis is the analyst's first task with his or her patients. No patient can open up to an analyst who is not open to him or her. The analyst must work through and resolve his own "defensive desire" to get rid of or to deflect objectionable or offensive defenses in order that he or she may analyze the meaning, purpose, and impact of the patient's defensive desire. It is crucial, for example, that the analyst not be put off—intimidated into masochistic passivity or provoked into sadistic activity—by the narcissistic defenses of a patient and not be frightened off by their coincident unconscious childhood needs.

When the analyst is centered in his or her selfness, he or she is then free to work openly with patients' self-centeredness. The analyst can then inquire freely into why the patient feels unacceptable except on grandiose grounds, without recourse to manipulation, moralizing, hostility, ingratiation, or rejection if the patient cannot at the moment move beyond his or her defensive desire. When analysts can accept their inevitable separateness and solitariness and can carry out such a free inquiry, they are then ready to meet the patient's true desire, that is, the patient's deep desire, however surrounded or suffused with defensiveness, to be accepted for his or her authentic selfness. This true desire must be met with acceptance and approval; here the analyst must not fail if serious harm to the analysis is to be prevented. If the analyst fails in this, the patient cannot grow, for he or she merely encounters the old way of relating. However, in the analytic work space of coparticipant inquiry, the patient can find a new way to relate to the analyst and can begin to fulfill his or her true desire for a more abundant life among other people.

CHAPTER 12

Coparticipant Transference Analysis

For the coparticipant analyst, as for all analysts, the concept of transference—the unconscious transfer of psychic experience from one interpersonal context to another—defines a central dimension of psychoanalytic inquiry, one that is critical for the in-depth therapeutic study of psychic suffering. Transference refers to the reliving of past experience in present interaction with others; that is, the present is misidentified as the past. One responds to others as though they were in some way significant figures of one's childhood. Transference (and countertransference) relatedness is thus marked by this irrational carryover of early feelings, attitudes, behaviors, fantasies, beliefs, and ideals. The coparticipant psychoanalytic situation is fundamentally a human relationship much like any other. The coparticipant analyst and his or her patient bring with them a unique and diverse set of motives and integrating tendencies. Thus, every transference pattern represents a unique therapeutic dynamic. Transference (and countertransference) patterns differ in emotional intensity, breadth of parataxic involvement, level of rationality (ranging on a continuum of psychic disturbance from mildly neurotic to delusionally psychotic), psychic significance, and in their representative dynamic themes.

In the clinical psychoanalytic situation, as in everyday life, one's experience comprises a complex, constantly shifting and continuously flowing amalgam of transferential and nontransferential relatedness. All interpersonal and intrapersonal processes represent dynamic combinations of these relational dimensions. Though separable conceptually, the experiential dimensions of transference-countertransference relatedness and the actual relationship (what is often called the "real relationship") are inevitably interpenetrating processes and in this sense clinically indivisible. This psychic complexity and attendant difficulty in disentangling the transferential from the nontransferential is one of the reasons for the relatively long time required for the psychoanalytic exploration and resolution of patients' difficulties in living.

Coparticipant inquiry, like participant and nonparticipant inquiry, emphasizes the curative significance of transference analysis; however, coparticipant inquiry is unique in viewing transference and countertransference as reciprocal and interpenetrating processes that are continuously active and interactive in the mutual formation of a coparticipant or intersubjective therapeutic field of psychoanalytic inquiry. In essence, transference and countertransference (defined here as the analyst's transference to his or her patient) form an interpersonal matrix of irrational experience. These two reciprocal processes, transference and countertransference, may be thought of as representing a co-created psychic dynamism—in Sullivan's terms, a "relatively enduring [and recurrent] pattern of energy transformations" (1953, p. 103). The clinical vicissitudes of this dynamic combination of parataxic experience are experienced and explored jointly by patient and analyst.

Coparticipant conceptions of transference and approaches to its analysis, as discussed previously (see especially chapters 1, 2, and 11), are unique in their radical view of transference and countertransference as *co-created and coanalyzed* parataxic experience. The analyst's personality is seen as a formative factor in all transferential relatedness. Countertransference is both shaped by and expressed in the transference, and, similarly, transference is both shaped by and expressed in the countertransference. In coparticipant analysis transference and countertransference are seen as clinical amalgams of self and situation, each deriving its full meaning in relation to its reciprocal.

According to this coparticipant approach to transference and countertransference, the analysis of countertransference is crucial to the analysis of transference and to a therapeutic understanding and working through of the patient's neurotic difficulties in living. Moreover, in coparticipant analysis, the patient is encouraged to be a coanalyst—to participate as fully as possible in the analysis of both transference and countertransference. This coparticipant approach to the psychoanalytic situation cuts across theoretical lines, reflecting new and converging developments in contemporary interpersonal psychoanalysis, intersubjective theory, self psychology, modern object relations, and in some forms of contemporary Freudian practice.

Since the coparticipant approach to transference and its analysis has already been addressed in several preceding chapters, I will here only review briefly some observations and hypotheses about the analysis of transference that I have found especially useful in therapy and that represent principles of coparticipant inquiry I articulated in chapters 1 and 2.

COUNTERTRANSFERENCE ANALYSIS IN THE ANALYSIS OF TRANSFERENCE

A critically important clinical implication of the coparticipant concept of transference and countertransference is that understanding the patient's personality inevitably involves understanding the analyst's personality. In other words, the analysis of countertransference is an integral aspect of transference analysis (and vice-versa).

For the coparticipant analyst transference relatedness represents an amalgam of the past and present, always incorporating in its evolving structure elements of the analyst's personality. That is to say, patients unconsciously shape their transferential tendencies to the contours of their analysts' personalities (and interpersonal vulnerabilities and necessities). Thus, a patient usually will unconsciously structure and express the same transference tendency differently with different analysts. For example, as pointed out in chapter 2, a patient will tailor his or her vengeful hostility to the unique vulnerability of his or her analyst. This will engender a different response from different analysts, which in turn will provoke a response tailored to the analyst's counterreaction, and so on. Transference thus moves into the present and toward the future as it simultaneously reaches back into the past.

Within the dyadic field of coparticipant inquiry patients' and analysts' personalities constantly influence each other's transferential relatedness. For example, when and how completely patients will express their transferential sexuality will depend on who their analysts are, what they value and believe, and how they relate to their own sexuality. Similarly, a patient's transference dependency will to some degree be shaped to conform to the analyst's unconscious needs and vulnerabilities. This same dependency would be expressed differently with different analysts, each time unconsciously tailored to the analyst's personality. In turn, different analysts will react differently, and again elicit a different reaction from the patient, and so on in expanding recursive complexity. Every analytic dyad generates its own unique transference-countertransference matrix.

Since in the coparticipant viewpoint countertransference contributes to the formation and clinical unfolding of transference, its analysis is considered relevant to the analysis of transference (and vice-versa). Thus, transference becomes a more complex, dyadic phenomenon than when seen from a monadic, nonparticipatory view of analysis. For example, in the nonparticipatory approach a patient's transference experience of curiosity is seen only as an expression of some endogenous dynamic (e.g., primal sexuality, infantile dependency, or "basic" hostility). As a result, other possible unconscious motivations (e.g., love, altruistic desire to help, or fearful ingratiation) that are interactionally linked to countertransference experience (e.g., the analyst's exhibitionism, loneliness, or desire for treatment) may be overlooked, and a more complex meaning of the patients' transference may be lost.

Coparticipant analysts usually focus on both their patient's and their own analytic experience, and the patient is encouraged to do the same. This characterizes the coparticipant path to the understanding of the patient's unconscious conflicts and problems in living. A non-coparticipant approach to transference and countertransference, even if relational in metapsychology, may limit or skew the analyst's understanding of the patient and himself or herself. In any event, it inevitably devitalizes the potential richness that a coparticipant approach promises. While other approaches may consider, for example, a secretly provocative patient's continual asking for advice simply transferential dependency, in a coparticipant inquiry the analyst's countertransference experience of being vaguely irritated with the patient would be included as subject of the inquiry, and thus the patient's unconscious transactional intent may come to light. From this point many more avenues for potential inquiry open up. The coparticipant inquiry into this transference-countertransference interaction—how the patient continually punishes her analyst with a false helplessness—may be initiated by either the patient or the analyst, depending on who, at the moment, is most ready.

Throughout the course of an analysis, the analyst's psyche is present with that of his or her patient's. Inevitably, the unconscious of the analyst and that of the patient intersect in the intersubjective spaces of the coparticipant field of therapy. For the coparticipant analyst transference and countertransference are interconnected processes that are then explored within a coparticipant field of shared experience and inquiry. In other words, transference analysis and countertransference analysis form integral aspects of one another. The coparticipant analytic field may thus be seen as a special instance of all human relatedness: a complex and ever-shifting dynamic of transference and countertransference, past and present, illusion and reality.

Analysis of the countertransference in the analysis of transference is important, not only because countertransference is built into the transference and thus integral to its analysis; it is as present analytically as transference and is thus available to patients' developing skill and interest in analyzing and understanding the nature of unconscious experience, their own and that of others. In a truly coparticipant inquiry, patients experience the analysis of countertransference as a natural extension of their expanding coparticipation in the analysis of their transference relatedness.

TRANSFERENCE AS A DYNAMIC STRUCTURE OF EXPERIENCE

All transference patterns represent a complex nexus of integrating tendencies (need), processes of anxiety, and security operations (defenses). Transference processes are in constant flux, whether the coparticipants are aware of them or not. Transference processes and patterns vary in their dynamic significance and clinical breadth, and their countless facets often shift unpredictably in and out of focus. Transference reactions may be triggered by an infinite variety of stimuli and appear in response to a great variety of interpersonal events or situations.

Transference is basically an adaptive effort to cope with new situations by generalizing from previous experience. One carries over the old and familiar to the new and unfamiliar, equating the present with the past. Transference is thus generalization gone wrong— a "pathological generalization," as Erwin Singer put it. It forms what Jean Piaget, the seminal Swiss developmental theorist, called an assimilative world schemata; however, one that asymmetrically ignores the individual's reciprocal need to also adjust to the environment in order to intelligently and adaptively interact with it.

All transference patterns, as noted previously, encompass a complex nexus of need, anxiety, and defenses, any one of which may emerge at any given moment. We crudely label transference experience as being this or that kind of transference in terms of its most salient characteristic (e.g., oedipal, narcissistic, mirroring, hostile, passive-dependent). In actuality, however, transference patterns represent very complex phenomena with multiple, perhaps innumerable, facets.

Transference and countertransference originate not in the regressive pull of the repetition compulsion, the blind instinctual need to repeat or to return to an earlier state. Rather, they arise from the dialectics of the interpersonal self's pull for security and the personal self's push for self-fulfillment. For coparticipant analysts, the meaning of transference and of repetitive behavior in general lies in the interpersonal dynamics of anxiety and the defensive operations of the self-system. The self-protective function of transference generalizations reflects the universal human need to secure a sense of interpersonal safety and predictability, that is, to avoid the threats anxiety and apprehension pose to the self.

Transference generalizations may be thought of as pathological attempts to perpetuate a rigidly uniform view of the world in which all is seen reductively in terms of one's unique life experience. For example, based on prior experience with cruel and critical parents, patients may see all people, including the analyst, as hostile and harsh. Specific early experiences are generalized into beliefs about the way the world is. The ways one's early significant others related are interpreted as typical of human nature. Through repression, dissociation, selective inattention, and other defensive operations, patients (and others) thus ignore or deny new experiences that contradict their transferred expectations and ensure the transferential similarity of new and old interpersonal situations. Life is what one has lived, rather than a set of new possibilities. This dialectic constitutes the work of psychoanalysis.

In Singer's (1965) coparticipant view, transference represents a defensive whitewash of one's unique history and experience; in transferential relatedness all people are seen as essentially alike. Through this leveling process, patients temper the threatening implications of their fury toward those who had actually hurt them. From this viewpoint, the traditional definition of transference and countertransference reactions as either positive or negative is irrational, for transferential relatedness aims at maintaining a fixed sameness in interpersonal experience and thus necessarily involves a rejection of the unique individuality of others and inevitably limits one's self-awareness. The defensive pull of the interpersonal self eclipses the forward push of the personal self.

Transference and countertransference manifest themselves not only in unconscious patterns of apprehension and anxiety but also in reenactments of earlier traumatizing experiences with others. Patients (and analysts) may pressure others, including their analytic copartners, in many nonverbal ways to behave or react the same way as the significant adults of the person's childhood. Thus, patients (or analysts) not only transferentially reexperience their earlier anxious experiences but also interactionally recreate them (Levenson 1972). Consequently, later life experiences can reinforce individuals' original transferential patterns, which are thus recreated over and over again. Transference, in this sense, becomes self-perpetuating, and a self-fulfilling prophecy.

TRANSFERENCE AND COUNTERTRANSFERENCE AS COMPLEX INTEGRALS OF LIFE EXPERIENCE

Transference and countertransference are open-ended and continually evolving dynamics, not static repetitions of early experiences. Formed in early childhood, transference patterns are more or less modified by subsequent experience. They are not static processes but are always in flux and to an extent include later experiences that have modified and reinforced the initial ones to some extent. Thus, in coparticipant inquiry transference represents the clinical expression of a complex characterological integral of life experience.

As Wolstein observes, transference processes "not only reproduce the old, they also reconstruct it in new and changing ways" (1954, p. 38). In this potential for repatterning lies, the possibility of analytic change and self-transformation. However, a person's developmental process may have reinforced his or her early transference patterns in subsequent life experience, making them more resistant to change. Regarding this point, Erwin Singer (1965) emphasizes that the greater the "number of situations the patient has encountered in his life which forced him to develop his particular system of beliefs . . . the more massively and early in his life the patient has encountered insistence on self-restriction, the more readily will he have developed once-and-for-all parataxic generalizations" (p. 265). Nevertheless, as previously noted, the open-ended nature of transference experience always carries a potential for analytic growth and personal transformation.

As I explained elsewhere (Fiscalini 1995b),

> Transference patterns and proclivities originally developed in early interpersonal relations with significant others are continually reconfigured or reinforced in myriad smaller or larger ways by subsequent interpersonal experiences. These elaborations and modifications, in turn, continually alter relationships with others (and experiences of them), leading to even further elaboration or modification of transference patterning. This dynamic spiral, of course, may move in either a positive or negative direction, leading in the extremes either to transference rigidity and personality constriction or to constructive expansion of one's personality. . . . Since transference represents an integral of life experience, its analysis consists of working through successive layers of complexly related developmental experience—working through, in other words, both the earliest pathogenetic experiences and the evolving defensive character traits, neurotic goals, and compensatory drives that are subsequently developed around them. (pp. 632–633)

TRANSFERENCE EXPRESSED THROUGH MULTIPLE MODALITIES

Transference and countertransference patterns manifest themselves in several different ways; analysts thus have many ways of observing or listening for transference experience.

Coparticipant analysts generally focus on verbal and behavioral (or interactional) indices of transference relatedness as analytic data. The primary sources of transference information for the analyst are the following communicative channels: (1) *direct or indirect verbal narratives,* which take two forms: (a) directly verbalized transferential feelings, thoughts, and wishes by the patient; and (b) inferred transference experience gleaned from patients' accounts of their relationships with their analysts or significant others. Closely related to this is (2) the *allusional,* or symbolic, form, that is, the use of indirect (displaced) communication in which patients talk about their relations with others and the world but are unconsciously alluding to some aspect of their relationship to and experience of the analyst or the analytic situation. Of course, most analysts, not just coparticipant ones, listen for these expressions of transference. In addition, there is (3) the *metaphoric* mode, as in dream processes and other expressive forms of primary process or prelogical communication. These preverbal processes are important sources of unconscious communication and understanding of transference and countertransference patterns. A closely related communicative modality is (4) *induced experience,* that is, the use of subjective countertransferential experience as an intuitive or empathic clue to the nature of the transference. This mode of listening or communication reflects the analyst's unconscious attunement to the patient's unconscious transference experience. Some analysts are more comfortable with this kind of unconscious communication (Bass 2001a); however, coparticipant analysts generally tend to be more open than noncoparticipant analysts to the therapeutic use of such modes of unconscious communication. Clearly, two people may share an empathic, parataxic bond that allows communication without words or through very primitive alogical symbolism. This wordless connection may be transitory and temporary or more enduring. Lastly, in addition to the just noted sources of information about transference, there are (5) the *transactive or enactive* aspects of transference relatedness.

Analysts and patients may prefer one communicative channel or listening modality over the others. For example, some analysts find that they work best with transactive data, whereas others may favor listening for allusions. Other analysts easily use all five communicative channels or some combination of them. The modality of transference communication a particular analyst focuses on may vary in accordance with his or her personal preferences and the psychological status of the patient, the current state of the analytic relationship, and the stage of the analysis.

Coparticipant analysts use both free association and focused association as methods of inquiry. In contrast to nonparticipant practitioners, they believe that a focused and detailed inquiry is more efficient than one following solely free association methodology. This detailed inquiry, traditionally directed to the analysis of extratransference in participant forms of inquiry, may also be applied to the exploration of transference and countertransference processes and patterns.

TRANSFERENCE AND COUNTERTRANSFERENCE AS ENACTIVE AND EXPERIENTIAL PHENOMENA

Transferential enactments (interpersonal transactions) characterize all analyses. By provoking reciprocal countertransference responses similar to those lived out in the patients' original pathogenic relations with their parents and other significant caretakers patients recreate and reenact their traumatic childhood relationships. As previously noted, patients can unconsciously pressure their analysts to react like the important people in their childhood. This fact has generally been interpreted in terms of the operation of projective identification (Klein 1948), as object-relational role responsiveness (Sandler 1976), and as the patient's interpersonal transformation of the analyst (cf. Levenson 1972, 1983).

According to the coparticipant perspective, analytic enactments result from the subtle and complex interplay of overlapping transference and countertransference processes (Grey and Fiscalini 1987). The coparticipant study of how analysts fit in with their patient's neuroses can prove informative and serve as a living source of knowledge about patients' transference experiences. These processes run reciprocally; that is, what is true for the coparticipant patient holds true for the coparticipant analyst who also enacts, as well as experiences, his or her transferential needs, anxieties, and self-protective defenses.

COPARTICIPANT INQUIRY AND EARLY EXPLORATION OF TRANSFERENCE

While Freud tolerated the "unobjectable positive transference" and emphasized the interpretive priority of the negative transference, most coparticipant analysts recommend the analysis of both positive and negative transference from the very beginning of a patient's treatment. Coparticipant analysts, particularly those of a more radical bent, believe that allowing the positive transference to intensify over a long period of time is therapeutically counterproductive. Wolstein, for example, warns that when analysts ignore the "first notes of transference distortion," they will allow it "to become a crescendo," and thereby they may compromise their therapeutic leverage by thus placing themselves "in the position of not being able to analyze it in full emotional force . . . because the patient will not have had any gradual introduction to the understanding of its manifestations" (1954, p. 58). Moreover, the tacit encouragement of impossible hopes implicitly nested in the positive transference may contribute to the iatrogenic development of narcissism and other pathological dependencies.

Though transference interpretation and inquiry may be more effective during analytic periods when transference resistance is minimal or when the patient's relationship with the analyst is relatively positive, coparticipant analysts usually interpret and inquire into transference experience, whether negative or positive, right from the start. Transference inquiry begins as soon as there is sufficient reason to question the possible transference meaning of patients' analytic relatedness. Most coparticipant analysts disagree with Freud's assertion that transference does not manifest itself at the very beginning of treatment and maintain instead that transference appears clinically, even if only in rudimentary forms, from the very first moments of an analysis. Coparticipant exploration of transference begins as soon as the analyst (or patient) has some clear sense of its occurrence; and its interpretation begins as soon as the analyst knows enough to coherently formulate significant aspects of the patient's transference relatedness. Such analytic activity, of course, is premised on the patient's demonstrated readiness and willingness to work in the transference. Though more radical coparticipant analysts tend to interpret or inquire into transference processes continuously and early, not all such analysts feel comfortable with such early intervention, preferring to wait and see how the analytic relationship shapes itself. Patients and analysts vary considerably in their readiness to work with transference and countertransference processes in an analysis.

In coparticipant inquiry there is no effort to systematically foster a regression to a transference neurosis. Regressive processes are, of course, duly noted by all coparticipant analysts, and transference, by definition, is a regressive phenomenon. Coparticipant analysts, however, do not generally attempt to induce regressive experiences but merely allow them to unfold. Many analysts, particularly those of a more conservative bent, think a highly interactive analytic stance interferes with the encouragement of therapeutic regression. However, most coparticipant analysts believe that analytic activity and an interactive analytic stance promote the full emergence of salient transference issues (Fiscalini 1994a).

EXPLORATION OF "HERE-AND-NOW" TRANSFERENCE, EXTRATRANSFERENCE, AND HISTORICAL EXPERIENCE IN COPARTICIPANT INQUIRY

Coparticipant analysts emphasize here-and-now transference inquiry but also work with extratransference and genetic—i.e., historical—experience.

The coparticipant analyst Edgar Levenson (1972, 1982a) maintains that the working through process is facilitated by the interpretive coordination—the pointing out of parallels—of transference, extratransference, and historical experience. Such interpretive patterning contributes significantly to patients' developing awareness of the major patterns of their behavior and experience. Further, insights gleaned in the exploration of any one of these central dimensions of relatedness may promote further understanding of the other domains of inquiry. Thus, for example, a new understanding of a particular pattern of one's parataxic involvement with one's spouse may stimulate early memories and lead to further insights about such history, or it may facilitate new insight into one's transference relatedness. Such interpretive connections can move in many directions and occur in complex combinations.

For coparticipant analysts, the analysis of the here-and-now transference, of the patient's shifting analytic experience and relatedness, is the major instrument of analytic insight. The focus of inquiry is on the interpretive and experiential exploration of the interactional patterns of transference and countertransference.

Transference is, of course, the primary source of analytic resistance, and it is also the medium for the analytic working through of one's difficulties in living. Transference interpretations—pointing out to patients what they are doing or seem to be experiencing *as* they are doing or experiencing it—inevitably carry an emotional immediacy and conviction not usually found in extratransference or historical interpretations, which deal with events at a distance. This explains the greater therapeutic efficacy of transference interpretations and inquiry. It is only in this domain of inquiry that patients' problems are analyzed as they emerge.

While the contemporary emphasis on here-and-now transference analysis has certain merits, an exclusive, one-sided focus on this domain and the corresponding neglect of extratransference and historical experience leaves patients feeling lost in the present, without a sense of historical continuity or a framework in which to comprehend the evolution and scope of their parataxic problems. Conversely, the recovery or reconstruction of the past without an experiential awareness of its impact upon one's present living seldom leads to therapeutic growth. Moreover, a neurotic character pattern or transference dynamic cannot be resolved by simply referring it to its historical origins, for later life experiences, involving pathological goals and defenses, have become part of this evolving pattern. Patients bring to the clinical psychoanalytic situation a complex, multifaceted defensive system that incorporates conflicting compensatory drives and defenses; it must be therapeutically unraveled, one strand at a time, beginning with the functional dynamics of its current adaptation.

Here-and-now transference analysis is the most alive form of psycho-analytic inquiry and the principal modality of therapeutic action; yet, as previously noted, genetic and extratransference inquiry are important in that they give the patient a sense of his or her own history and developmental path. They also provide an important source of ancillary information, offering a more rounded picture of the patient as a person and confirming transference interpretations.

Extratransference inquiry is part of all analytic work, particularly with those patients who seem unable to address the transferential "me-you" relationship. The coparticipant inquiry moves back and forth, from one domain of inquiry to another. One of the skills of a good analyst is knowing when to move from one to another aspect of the inquiry, intuiting when it is best to work in the transference or the extratransference or with the patient's history. To sum up, most coparticipantly oriented analysts emphasize the analytic primacy of transference and countertransference inquiry while also acknowledging the importance of inquiry and interpretation of the patient's extra-analytic relationships, past and present.

In the initial stages of the treatment of some seriously disturbed or anxious patients it may be important to concentrate on working with extratransference experience. Often narcissistic or deeply disturbed patients, given their undeveloped sense of self and separateness, initially find it impossible to work in the transference. Transference analysis is often experienced initially by such patients as an expression of criticism or blame or, ironically, as an example of the analyst's narcissism. Extratransference data may be an important source of information about patients' problems in living, and it may serve to confirm (or disconfirm) transference hypotheses. Extratransference interpretations may anchor patients' understanding of themselves and their problems within a broader social context.

THE WORKING ALLIANCE

The psychoanalytic process is arduous, and the rigors of coparticipant inquiry are daunting, requiring a considerable commitment of time, financial resources, and emotional energy. More important, coparticipant inquiry demands a commitment to face oneself and one's deepest desires and fears, to reveal oneself to another and to bear the anxieties of trusting someone. In addition, there are the analytic terrors of self-transformation and of going beyond previous limits of acceptable consciousness and into the unknown. Patients thus must be willing to bear the shame, rage, sorrow, and other painful emotions that accompany honest self-inquiry and self-knowledge. To sustain such a coparticipant encounter and analytic endeavor requires the development of a solid working alliance.

The establishment of a working or therapeutic alliance—the conscious and unconscious coparticipant commitment of patient and analyst to work together as steadily and collaboratively as possible—need not rest on the suggestive basis of an "unobjectionable positive transference." An effective working alliance is usually based on a variety of factors that promote the formation of a strong coparticipant tie between patient and analyst. This facilitative aspect of the analytic relationship we call the working alliance involves all those facets or qualities of one's character (whether one is patient or analyst) that work toward effective coparticipant analysis, and it reflects the play and interplay of several factors.

Before reviewing these factors, I would like to note that an effective working alliance between patient and analyst is premised upon a good fit between them; in other words, they have to be compatible in sensitivity, transference needs and defensive systems, general world view, and analytic temperament. Such a psychological fit would provide the working basis for a mutually empathic, yet challenging coparticipant exploration of the patterns of transference and countertransference characteristic of a given psychoanalytic dyad. In a sense, I am describing here the qualities of "coparticipant analyzability," *the capacity of analyst and analysand to analyze and be analyzed by the other*.

Not all patients and analysts can work well with one another. No matter how similar in outlook and "feel" any particular pairing of analyst and patient may be, too intense or negative an immediate transference or countertransference may be too explosive or emotionally intense to provide sufficient emotional space to build a working alliance. In such instances, it may prove best for patient and analyst to review the nature and course of their mutual incompatibilities and possibly reconsider whether they have a good enough fit to allow the necessary work to take place. If there is enough of a therapeutic connection to allow work with the initial transference or countertransference difficulties, to allow the seeds of future collaboration to be sown, the patient and analyst may find themselves in a tight and uncomfortable and even volatile but nonetheless promising *coparticipant fit*.

Patients and analysts sometimes defensively choose each other on the basis of shared or converging resistances, forming a collusive partnership in which there is a tacit agreement to avoid or abort any inquiry that would create anxiety and disrupt either coparticipant's defensive harmony. These are the analyses that essentially don't touch the deeper personal pain each coparticipant suffers, nor the joy that a more challenging treatment would provide. In such an analytic relationship, the essential patterns of transference and countertransference remain unknown and unrevealed. The therapeutic alliance is essentially distorted into a therapeutic misalliance.[1]

I have found that achieving a solid and effective working alliance is based on a variety of personal and interpersonal factors, including the effects of the therapeutic process I call living through and the activation of what is often called basic trust, that is, the consensually valid (i.e., nontransferential) generalization of the experience of interpersonal tenderness. In addition, the working alliance requires rational hope and expectations of help, clinical courage, and the many inner resources constituting the proactive, self-generating and self-moving strivings and capacities of the personal self.

ON TRANSFERENCE DISTORTION AND INTERPRETATION

In recent years, some analysts with a perspectivistic and relativistic epistemology have questioned the concept of transference as distortion. In their post-Freudian critiques of the "blank screen" concept, Gill (1982a, 1983) and Hoffman (1983) emphasize that transference is invariably related to here-and-now analytic interaction and always includes *plausible* interpretations of the analyst's experience. Transference is defined as selectivity in awareness or rigidity in perception, rather than as distorted misattribution. Transference is also seen to function like a Geiger counter, with past experience sensitizing one to possible meanings that others might overlook or find insignificant.

Critical of authoritarian concepts of the objective analyst, Hoffman, Gill, Levenson, Racker, Stolorow, and Wolstein, among other theorists of a broadly coparticipant sensibility, reject the notion that the analyst is the arbiter of analytic reality. For analysts of a strongly hermeneutic bent, such as Hoffman (1983, 1992) and Stern (1997), analytic truth and meaning are socially constructed. The relativistic sensibility of analysts of the participant-observer paradigm, particularly those of the interpersonal school, anticipated this new analytic epistemology. These analysts, like coparticipant analysts, hold a democratic concept of analytic authority. Sullivan, for example, spoke of consensual validation—truth as social agreement—thus placing a culturally and interpersonally determined concept of truth at the interpretive center of psychoanalytic practice. Truth and interpretive self-knowledge of both patient and analyst are seen as provisional, always open to revision.

For coparticipant analysts, interpretive or narrative truth derives from social consensus and interpretive authority is shared by patient and analyst; thus, neither partner's truth rules. Though interpretations of transference and countertransference ultimately are social constructions, they originate in private and uniquely individual experiences, in "asocial" constructions, as it were. They are both personally formed and interpersonally formulated.

The perspectivistic epistemologies of many contemporary or postmodern analysts emphasize the inherent ambiguity of clinical events. However, our coherence theories of truth (which are implicit in relativistic epistemologies) are always circumscribed by some correspondence to reality, although we may not be able to know that reality except through our constructions of it.

In contrast to the psychic relativism of some coparticipant analysts, others emphasize the realism of immediate experience. Though these two varieties of coparticipant inquiry do not share similar epistemologies, they share a common criticism of the classical, nonparticipant paradigm of psychoanalytic praxis. These contemporary trends represent an argument against analytic authoritarianism as well as a critique of the classical concepts of analytic impersonality and anonymity.

The concept of the analytic situation as an interpersonal therapeutic field and of analytic interpretation as socially constructed meaning does not, however, require a rejection of the concept of transference as irrationality or distortion. Transference reactions may be anchored in patients' plausible or even current experiences of their analysts' unconscious minds; however, they are also invariably distorted, in some way shaped by past experience.

Transference distortion is implicit in the perceptual rigidity and attentional selectivity that frequently characterizes transference relatedness. The analyst, as Gill (1982a,b) and Hoffman (1983) rightly emphasize, is rigidly seen in certain set ways. The patient may focus rigidly on a particular quality in the analyst's attitude or behavior and may exaggerate its pervasiveness or prominence in the analyst's total relatedness. Distorted relatedness is also inherent in patients' transferentially exaggerated responses to their analysts' analytic coparticipation. Patients may plausibly or validly sense, for example, anger or disapproval in their analyst's attitude but exaggerate or misjudge its emotional amplitude, motivation, unconscious meaning, or dynamic significance in the analyst's personality. In other words, transference distortion manifests itself in *miscontextualizing* analytic data.

Though transference may, as Hoffman (1983) suggests, operate like a Geiger counter, shaping a selective sensitivity to certain facets of the analyst's personality and subjectivity, it also operates to inappropriately emphasize this facet over others equally important. The analyst is, as it were, interpreted in terms of a *narrow or reductive context*. Transference distortion is also implicit in the use of what may be called *improbable contexts*; that is, the analyst's behaviors and attitudes may be attributed to irrelevant or unlikely reference frames or contexts. For example, the patient may plausibly interpret an analyst's repeated clearing of his or her throat at a certain juncture in a session as a sign of restive boredom or unconscious anger, when in reality the analyst is simply recovering from a cold, or, even if irritated, bored, or anxious that these feelings are related to the patient in more complex or different ways than the patient imagines. The concept of transference as distortion is implicit in the common observation that there are always varying *degrees* of plausibility whenever clinical events are interpreted.

Transference distortion is perhaps most clearly exemplified in the emotional carryover of childhood responsiveness in analytic experience of the self. It is not unusual for patients to accurately appraise facets of their analysts' personalities (their hostility, contempt, anxiety, dependency, warmth, etc.) but often these same patients distort the emotional import of this, experiencing their analysts' traits with all the intensity and meaning involved in their childhood experience of their parents and other significant adults. While it is not surprising that the analyst is similar in significant respects to the parents of the patient's childhood, the patient is no longer *that child, except in transference distortion.* The distortion of the transference reaction thus lies in the meaning or significance attributed to the analyst's attitude and behavior, in reacting as though the analyst had the same power and significance in one's life that one's parents had in one's childhood. Transference distortion is located ultimately in the transfer of self experience.

Clearly, from a coparticipant perspective the concept of transference (or countertransference) distortion as pure illusion or pure projection is questionable (though at times transference reactions may be, in clinical fact, almost entirely imaginary or illusory projections). Nevertheless, when viewed more broadly, the concept of transference as distortion seems clinically valid. The unresolved relationships of one's past inevitably structure, limit, and complicate—in other words, distort—one's present relatedness.

In sum, transference or countertransference distortions define a continuum of irrational or illusory relatedness, ranging from slight skews in analytic experience to gross, psychotic-like warps in analytic relatedness. Transference or countertransference symbolizations, as they begin to take form, always reach out to the present while simultaneously reaching into the past. Transference and countertransference represent a dialectical interplay of present and past, fact and fiction. The past shapes itself to fit the present as that present is shaped by the past.

INTERPRETATION AND COPARTICIPANT INQUIRY

Coparticipant analysts do not offer transference interpretations as statements of a universal metapsychological truth. Rather, they view interpretive formulations as working hypotheses—provisional or partial truths—that inevitably require the patient's interpretive participation for their elaboration, modification, and final acceptance or rejection. Sullivan, for example, was wary about the possible misuse and overuse of analytic interpretations. He sardonically reminds us that "the supply of interpretations, like that of advice, greatly exceeds the need for them" (1940, p. 187). Sullivan maintained that all interpretations should be tested by the *laws of adequacy and exclusivity;* that is, we should ask whether an interpretation covers the relevant data and if so, whether it is the most plausible (best) hypothesis available. Sullivan thought that if interpretations could not meet these two tests, they should not be offered. Like contemporary coparticipant analysts, Sullivan always regarded interpretations as working hypotheses.

Consistent with their democratic, egalitarian perspective, coparticipant analysts view interpretation as a collaborative process. They encourage analytic mutuality and regard the patient as an active, psychoanalytic copartner rather than as a passive recipient of wisdom. As Sullivan (1954) commented sardonically, the idea that analysts, from their "acquired divinity, can tell a person what is the matter, ought really to be adjourned" (p. 211). As noted earlier, in coparticipant inquiry, analytic interpretations are viewed as provisional hypotheses, partial truths, that require the patient's interpretive coparticipation for their completion and confirmation. Many coparticipant analysts, in fact, evaluate the therapeutic efficacy of an interpretation on the basis of its ability to facilitate a deepening of transference inquiry rather on whether or not it provides metapsychological truth.

Coparticipant analysts vary in how subjectively certain or comprehensive they believe they must be in their formulative understandings before sharing them in interpretive questions or statements. Some coparticipant analysts are comfortable initiating the interpretive process with highly speculative interpretive comments or questions; others are more conservative. Generally, they consider it analytically important to encourage patients to formulate their own interpretive understanding of themselves.

Psychoanalytic interpretations are intended to help bring to awareness dissociated or repressed experience and motivation. Curative insight, however, does not come from one single clarifying analytic interpretation but rather from many repeated interpretations, each focused on one or another of the numerous facets of the patient's problems in living.

Interpretation is an art, as any analyst can attest. Interpretations may be offered in countless ways, as questions, comments, exclamations, selective repetitions of the patient's words, a relevant story, as well as in more formal interpretive statements, and so on. Adapting interpretations to the psychic needs of the patient should not, however, be achieved at the expense of the analyst's authenticity and his or her unique ways of self-expression.

UNIQUENESS IN ANALYTIC WORK

Because of the individuality and complexity of any single psychoanalysis, rules regarding transference inquiry or interpretation require many exceptions and qualifications. This is, in part, why the practice of psychoanalysis is an art as well as a science. There is no blueprint for the therapeutic sequence and timing of transference inquiry and interpretation or for extratransference interpretations and historical reconstructions; they are impossible to predict. Furthermore, interpretive guidelines should never substitute for clinical intuition or abrogate the free play of immediate analytic experience, of clinical directness and spontaneity.

Patients add to this psychoanalytic complexity because they use their acquired psychoanalytic self-knowledge in highly individual ways that are impossible to predict. Coparticipant analysts emphasize that all analyses represent unique sets or series of coparticipant processes that are ultimately dependent upon the unique qualities of the personalities making up each analytic dyad. Coparticipant psychoanalysis is a unique and highly individualized form of treatment and arguably more diverse in its practice than most other analytic approaches. It reflects theoretical and clinical pluralism and does not lend itself to codified rules.

CHAPTER 13

Living Through

The therapeutic action of psychoanalysis—the working through of patterns of irrational living—derives not simply from interpretation, as classically thought, but, more basically, from the experiential *living through* of these patterns in new ways, that is, by the formation, not just formulation, of new experience (Fiscalini 1988). This holds true for the successful resolution of all neurotic patterns of living. The working through of unmet yearning and defensive characterology requires that both aspects of neurosis—unlived need and defensive self-protection—be experientially lived through in new and different ways in the immediate personal relationship between analyst and patient.[1] Instead of relating, for example, to shamed, spoiled, and shunned aspects of the patient with familiar defensiveness and anxiety the analyst relates, authentically and spontaneously, to the patient's neurotic functioning in new, unexpected, and experientially corrective ways. The living through process is particularly crucial in working through the early preverbal experiential roots of patients' (and analysts') anxieties and difficulties in living.

The experiential living through of psychopathology, unlike its narrative interpretation, is not a technical process and thus cannot be consciously initiated by the analyst. This new reconstructive experience is made possible by the analyst (or patient) via his or her coparticipation as a new interpersonal object. It is neither planned nor role-played in Alexander's sense of a corrective emotional experience (Alexander and French 1946). Rather, it emerges spontaneously and authentically from the personal and relational being of the analyst (and patient) as he or she encounters and engages the patient's (and his or her own) neurosis and narcissism. And the patient may also coparticipantly serve as a new interpersonal object for the analyst in some unresolved or novel aspect of his or her living.

Living through refers to the reconstructive experience derived relationally from the inadvertent and unsought new, more mature, and relatively unconflicted interpersonal interactions between patient and analyst. Living through simply takes place because the analyst or the patient is who he or she is *as a person* and has nothing to do with a particular chosen analytic stance.

Like the personal relationship, the technical analytic relationship always reflects the personality of the analyst. Though traditionally the analyst was assumed to maintain a certain desirable anonymity during the analysis, that notion is actually based on the misconception that it is possible to separate technique from personality. Singer (1965), Goz (1975), and Bass (2001a,b), among a growing number of analysts, comment on the impossibility of avoiding self-revelation in meaningful analytic work. Even if not self-disclosing, the coparticipant analyst inevitably reveals significant dimensions of his or her personality in the intimate inquiry of psychoanalysis. The analyst may consciously or unconsciously attempt to hide behind an analytic persona. This, of course, limits the potential for intimacy and the coparticipatory possibilities of the inquiry. Ironically, the analyst, in this very choice, reveals his or her fearfulness and blocks a conjoint, and potentially fruitful, inquiry into this aspect of his or her personality.

The personality of the analyst contributes critically to the development of the trust and rapport necessary for the patient (and analyst) to talk, listen, and work freely and openly. Only when patients feel empathically known and personally respected can they entrust themselves to the analyst's understanding and accept unwanted information about themselves Bromberg (1980a), for example, emphasizes that psychoanalytic change depends upon the therapeutic formation of a presyntaxic transitional or bridging structure, a deep empathic bond that permits the patient to "partially suspend the operation of the self-system and 'take in' the analyst's rational attitude towards him [or her]" (p. 244). According to Bromberg, "This therapeutic regression is not pathological. It is not a return to symbiosis, but the recreation of. . . the presymbolic bond" (p. 245) that is rooted in very early experiences of tenderness. The personal relationship plays a vital, though secondary, curative role in facilitating the development of a therapeutic alliance. However, this general facilitative effect of the personal relationship is distinct from its primary and specific curative effects.

The central analytic issues of both patient and analyst are always lived out in their immediate relationship, either in the transference-countertransference matrix, further reinforcing neurotic and narcissistic experience, or in the living through process. They may be lived through—repetitively and consistently lived newly and differently—giving both experiential authority to interpretive work and providing curative experience in direct relational form. For example, an analyst's personal (i.e., technically unintended) ability to consistently relate to and be with his or her patient's defensive omnipotent striving in a nondefensive and developmentally appropriate way differs significantly from the pathogenic anxiety and defensiveness the patient encounters in interactions with significant others. In my view, this new way of relating is instrumental in freeing the patient's ability to try out and seek confirmation for new ways of relating that spring from a more centered personal self. These issues cannot be fully worked through if they are not lived through in a new and more mature manner in the immediate analytic relationship.

Levenson (1982a,b) states that the power of the psychoanalytic process may lie in *what is said about what is done* (between analyst and patient), and Tenzer (1983) adds *it is what is said about what is done while it is being done* (p. 327). These are cogent points, but in my view *what is done about what is said, or what is done while what is said is being said* is equally crucial. Merton Gill (1982a) asserts that the analyst provides a new interpersonal experience in the very act of making an interpretation. Levenson (1972, 1982a,b) also emphasizes that interpretations are a form of interpersonal participation and as such carry pragmatic (behavioral) as well as semantic impact. In contrast to Gill, he focuses on the countertransference potential of interpretive activity. The interpretive act may, as Gill asserts, provide a new or reconstructive interaction. When it does, however, it is only one of the many ways and contexts in which this new interaction is lived out.

Analysts provide new interpersonal experience, or its possibility, not simply by the fact of interpreting but by the how and what of it and also in many other interventions and ways of being with patients, for example, by the way they listen, by how and when they ask questions, and so on. The coincident living through of an interpretive issue takes place across the social and contextual span of the analytic inquiry. It often is lived through during the focal analysis of other interpretive themes. The significant psychic issue that is being lived through may have a great deal or very little to do with the verbalized analytic theme of the moment.

THE LIVING THROUGH PROCESS AND CURATIVE ACTION

The living through process—the relational generating of new and curative experience—achieves therapeutic significance in two ways: (1) directly, as reconstructive relational experience, and (2) dialectically, as an integral aspect of the interpretive process, experientially confirming verbal formulation and enriching, elaborating, or modifying interpretive work.

The dynamic relation between interpretation and the personal relationship can be conceptualized as representing a dialectic between coexisting interpretive (narrative) and experiential dimensions of analysis. The immediately experienced relationship between patient and analyst can interpretively elaborate and amend as well as experientially confirm the interpretive work (while simultaneously disconfirming the patient's transference expectations). Alternatively, it may experientially contradict it. The analyst may countertransferentially relive the neurotic conflict with the patient, even though providing a valid interpretation of the patient's problems. The experienced relationship then contradicts the interpretive understanding; as a result, therapeutic change is stalled until one of the coparticipants is able to live through the issue in a new, nontransferential way. Even if the analyst accurately understands and interprets a patient's neurotic dynamics, change only occurs after the analyst has repeatedly interacted with the patient, across a number of analytic contexts, in a nonneurotic way that experientially affirms (and informs) the interpretive work.

The curative importance of the living through process in its direct role is often unappreciated in analytic work with patients' problems and personalities. What takes place relationally between the patient and his or her analyst experientially informs the patient about his or her specific difficulties and about new interpersonal possibilities and ways of being. This can bring about representational repatterning and therapeutic changes in the patient's defensive character structure that may be mediated by various syntaxic (logical thinking) and presyntaxic (alogical) cognitive processes, often operating in complex combination. The direct curative effects of the living through process may be brought about via insight or through other learning processes, such as operant conditioning, classical conditioning, social learning processes, modeling and identification processes, trial-and-error learning, desensitization or deconditioning processes, etc. Several of these learning processes may operate simultaneously, and change may or may not be accompanied by conscious insight. Often, change occurs silently and unconsciously, without either coparticipant being aware of the process initially. Not infrequently, the analyst or patient may ascribe psychoanalytic change to factors or dynamics that, though therapeutically important, are not the reasons for the patient changing.

Patients not only compulsively and unconsciously attempt to repeat pathological patterns of relatedness—to transform the analyst, as Levenson (1972) puts it. They also try to engage the analyst in new and constructive integrations to transform themselves. while they seek to repeat or perpetuate old, familiar kinds of relational experience, they also search for new ways of relating and new kinds of experience in an effort to change themselves. This drive for mental health, as Sullivan (1953) called it, characterizes all patients, and it constitutes an essential impetus for the living through process.

Over sixty-five years ago, the orthodox English psychoanalyst Edward Glover speculated that "in the deeper pathological states, a prerequisite of the efficiency of interpretation is the attitude, the true unconscious attitude of the analyst to his patients" (1937, p. 372). Glover is right though his insight is too limited; to be therapeutic, interpretive insight requires the experiential validation of the living through process, for *all* patients, whatever the nature or developmental level of their psychic conflicts or deficits.

The personal relationship is always there, and it always carries direct, albeit implicit (experiential), interpretive significance. Even when a salient issue is not addressed narratively, it may be resolved on the basis of what takes place in the relationship between patient and analyst. Often, the living through process is directly curative in subtle ways and about subtle issues that may not come up interpretively despite their importance in the patient's life. For example, a patient may develop a genuine sense of humor, a spiritual or philosophical perspective, a livelier sense of curiosity, playfulness, a more alive sense of being, and an increased sense of self-worth, and so on as a result of the reconstructive experience derived relationally from repeated *new* interpersonal interactions with the analyst.

The question arises what kind of therapeutic relationship characterizes an analysis if important psychic issues of the patient are not addressed narratively (interpretively). Is this a sign of counterresistance or counter-transference or a question of the analyst's inexperience or incompetence? Or is it a sign of the patient's resistance? Of course, any or all of the above may prove true in any particular instance. Nevertheless, not all dynamic issues are necessarily addressed narratively in any given analysis. An important problem of the patient may be lived through and worked through relationally while other more pressing or immediate ones are the subject of focused interpretive inquiry. Thus, a particular problem may not require explicit interpretive attention. After all, interactions having bearing on many other issues go on during the analysis of any interpretive issue. Several important psychic issues may be lived through concurrently, although one or another is usually in the narrative foreground at any particular moment in an analysis.

Although important issues can get worked through without formal interpretive attention, I don't think that is the way it usually works. If the patient is appropriately understood in his or her singularity (significant specifics), the salient psychic issues usually will have been addressed narratively as well as lived through experientially. Clearly, profound and enduring psychoanalytic change requires significant understanding, interpretive and experiential, of the patient by the analyst (and vice versa). The processes of self-understanding and self-transformation also demand certain resources or capacities of the patient. In my experience, the awareness, however rudimentary or reluctant, of psychic disorder and suffering accompanied by a desire to change, the ability for psychic work (see Antonovsky 1985), basic hope and trust, and, last but not least, courage have proven particularly important.

Witenberg (1981) observes that "the most common belief is that interpretations are curative. Those analysts who have asked patients what was meaningful in the 'good session' frequently find that the patients have gained self-esteem in ways that had not been intended" (p. 15). Patients' reports of having been deeply affected or changed by something unintended by the analyst or by some seemingly trivial or isolated analytic interaction or intervention may actually be screen memories or metaphors for some consistent and curatively significant set of new interpersonal experiences in the living through process. These findings reflect, in my view, the core of truth in Alexander's (1961; Alexander and French 1946) much maligned concept of the "corrective emotional experience"—that *we, as analysts, cure as much by who and how we are as by what we say.*

In psychoanalytic treatment, the analyst's unconscious or preconscious ability to relate in a significantly different and nonneurotic way to the patient's history of spoiled and shamed experience and behavior forms the unconscious curative foundation (and limit) of his or her ability to work successfully with his or her patient's problems in living. Much of a patient's opportunity to work through his or her early unmirrored or falsely mirrored experiences lies in the analyst's ability to consistently relate in developmentally "good enough" ways to the needs of the patient. For example, the therapeutic efficacy of analysts of predominantly narcissistic patients is determined by their ability to emotionally connect with and nonanxiously relive with their patients both the patients' dissociated narcissistic yearnings and their reciprocal need to relinquish their early grandiosity, as these reciprocal needs emerge in the analytic inquiry and interaction.

In the living through process, the analyst relates both to the patient's neurotic ways of relating learned earlier in life *and* to his or her potentials and possibilities for intimacy, individuation, and authentic living. Essentially, the analyst empathically mirrors and validates the patient's reciprocal needs for *both* unconditional and conditional approval as these are interpretively addressed in the narrative domain and interactionally lived out in the experiential domain of the analysis.

Appreciating the curative centrality of the living through process is, of course, *not* the same as attempting to parent the patient or to try to fulfill a conventional social, or even sensual, role for the patient—to substitute for life, in other words. One of the most important experiences in the living through process is that patients may have their need to be experimental and flexible experientially affirmed and validated. Generalizing from their therapeutic experience, they can make use in everyday life of what Pearce and Newton (1963) have called alternate validation. That is, the patient becomes able to use an increasingly wider range of validating "self-objects" and in this way expand his or her interpersonal possibilities. In other words, the living through process, in addition to its other properties, functions as a catalyst. By living through new experiences with the analyst, the patient becomes increasingly able to attempt new forms of relating with others.

By emphasizing the importance of the living through process, I mean to underscore that psychoanalytic inquiry inevitably involves a deep, personal relationship whose interactional properties determine its curative potential. Psychoanalysis, at its very foundation, is a human relationship, not a quasi-medical situation, and that relationship in itself is therapeutically pivotal.

The analyst's new ways of relating to the patient are not attempts to reparent the patient but show the analyst's respect for and connection with the patient's personal growth needs and his or her unique range of personal and interpersonal possibilities. This, I believe, forms the core of the analyst's centered and nonneurotic relatedness. When this way of relating to the patient is lived through over and over again, it eventually becomes an integral part of the patient's experience and can in turn be lived out with significant others in his or her everyday life. Central issues may be lived through relationally even if they are not narratively addressed. These, for example, may include the patient's striving for autonomy, fears of separateness and yearnings for openness and relatedness, desires for sensual and sexual pleasure, the need to accept human imperfection, limitation, and ordinariness; and the patient's drive for fulfillment of his or her unique individuality.

The living through process is crucially important in the working through of very early, learned fears and anxious patterns of experience that verbal interpretations often don't seem to reach in any affectively significant way. The living through process encompasses two relational therapeutic processes hypothesized by post-Freudians as especially significant in the treatment of severe personality disturbance: Kohut's (1984) transmuting internalization and Modell's (1978) elaboration of Winnicott's concept of the holding environment. Both of these curative processes represent delimited, though important, aspects of the broader process of living through, which is curatively pivotal in the working through and analytic resolution of very early learned core "narcissistic" difficulties. The repatterning of infantile and primitive shamed and spoiled experience requires a lengthy process of repetitively living through these issues and thus a prolonged period of analysis. It is this therapeutic requirement that often underlies the lengthy analyses needed for extensive personality change.

The living through process is essential in the reintegration of certain core needs for mirroring approval; only this relational process can provide the experiential acceptance that allows the patient to reclaim these needs as fully human and free to be expressed. Often it is the lengthy and repeated living through of the patient's interpersonal self in a new and accepting way that allows the patient to develop a central and enduring sense of being acceptable and lovable. Only after extensive repetitions can this therapeutic process become firmly established in the patient's psyche.

RELATIONSHIP, EXPERIENCE, AND THERAPEUTIC INTERACTION

Behind their defensive masks patients hide a pervasive sense of themselves as being wrong or bad or not acceptable in their unique selfhood; that is, they suffer from a core deficit in self-esteem. The therapeutic correction of this deeply imprinted and generalized self-loathing requires a lengthy process of living through these attitudes and feelings about the self. This process cannot be rushed and must repeatedly cover many different analytic contexts. It is this relational process, rather than formulative interventions, that ultimately touches the patient most deeply. And good enough time must be granted for this process to lead to solid, enduring change in these early damaged aspects of the psyche.

Patients need the deep, unconscious approval and acceptance of the analyst as it is revealed relationally in numerous analytic interactions. Living through and working through very early learned anxieties takes a very long time; to expect otherwise reflects, I believe, a countertransferential fear of deep involvement with the patient's psyche, a fear of one's own neurotic desires and anxieties, and a denial of psychic vulnerability. To expect that human change does not require years of hard work is simply to reveal one's personal despair and nihilism, no matter how it might be rationalized (for example, as an interest in therapeutic effectiveness, cost-efficiency, etc.). What makes an analysis successful is that the patient lives through early unapproved relational states with a "centered enough" analyst.

Of course, this is not to deny the obvious importance of interpretive work and of inquiry in general, but it must be emphasized that psychoanalytic inquiry is based on and requires a profound personal relationship that is itself curatively significant. Fairbairn (1958) emphasizes that the patient learns from what happens "between the patient and the analyst as persons." (p. 379). The analyst's personality inevitably reveals itself regardless of the methodology used in the analysis, and it is this factor that is critical in bringing about psychoanalytic change.

The living through process accounts for those analytic cures or successful outcomes that could not be predicted from other indices of the patient's analytic coparticipation; it may also explain why cure or therapeutic change does not occur where there seems to be an accurate or highly plausible interpretive understanding of the patient's problems and dynamics, and the analysis seems to proceed properly in a formal sense. It seems to me, in these instances the analyst does not or cannot unconsciously live through or connect emotionally and nonverbally with the patient's early needs for boundless cherishing or adoring or with his or her need for limits. The analyst, in other words, may not be able to emotionally connect with or meet crucial aspects of the patient's need to resume the developmental process of the self-respecting child, to relationally transform spoiled and shamed experience into self-respecting ways of living. For example, the analyst may not be able to connect with a patient's early sense of expansiveness, transferential idealized love, or the patient's individual strivings for autonomy and separateness. Only the analyst's ability to authentically live through patients' problems in new and different ways carries the *emotional* truth or conviction for the patient that new, life-affirming ways of living and being are possible.

The living through process, whether in its dialectic or direct curative role, consists of two interrelated phases or steps. First, the analyst relates to the patient's neurotic interpersonal patterns in ways that consistently contradict transferential expectation (or provocation). Thus, this aspect of the living through process is characterized by the patient's repeating old patterns, with the analyst consistently relating to them in a new way. The patient lives this through on an experiential level. The new interpersonal interaction in this partly old and partly new relationship (that is, the analyst new in his or her way but the patient old in his or hers) is repeated over and over, usually over a relatively long period of time and across a variety of analytic contexts. At some crucial point—highly individual, complexly determined, and difficult to predict—the patient attempts *new*, nontransferential ways of being more in line with his or her actual needs. The analyst continues to respond in ways that, for the patient, are new and different, that is, unlike those of other significant figures, past and present. This completes the cycle. There is now a fully new interpersonal interaction, with the patient having both the immediate experience of psychically surviving the anxiety of living out previously forbidden or unknown ways of thinking and feeling, and the prelogical experience of consistently new responses to his or her old and new perceptions and behaviors. In this second aspect of the living through process the analyst plays an important affirming or validating role. When this complex set of interactions is lived through repeatedly in a relatively consistent way, psychic repatterning or self-transformation occurs, sometimes formulated (i.e., accompanied by conscious insight) and sometimes not.

The process of self-transformation in psychoanalysis is a highly complex phenomenon mediated by several learning processes at various levels of awareness. The specific experiential effects of the living through process, whether in its dialectic or direct role, are necessary, though not sufficient, for analytic change. Also necessary are the bonds of empathy and trust that contribute crucially to the patient's ability to incorporate the new interpersonal interactions of the living through process as reconstructive interpersonal experience. Curatively pivotal, too, is the patient's immediate experience of the living through process.

LIVING THROUGH AND COPARTICIPATION

As a coparticipant dyadic process, living through moves in both analytic directions. In other words, it applies equally and symmetrically to patient and analyst. What has been said of the patient's coparticipation can also be said for that of the analyst. Patient and analyst forge a personal, coparticipant relationship within which they reciprocally and continuously impact upon each other's experience. Just as the analyst plays a curative role as a new interpersonal other ("object") for the patient, so, too, the patient plays a curative role as a new interpersonal other for the analyst.

Just as analysts, by virtue of the way they relate to their patients (including the pragmatics of their interpretations), create the possibility of fostering or introducing new experience or behavior, so patients may, by virtue of who they are and the way they relate, foster the development of new attitudes and abilities in the analyst.

The magnitude of the direct or dialectical curative impact of this bidirectional coparticipant process depends on the character and maturity of the dyadic coparticipants and on the compatibility of their personalities. In some cases, living through carries the major part of the therapeutic action of psychoanalysis and in others far less, but it is operative in all. It is one of the most overlooked ways in which the patient, without consciously trying or intending to, impacts positively on the analyst.

By virtue of his or her way of relating and interacting, the patient may foster the analyst's development of new ways of being and relating, for example, the development of greater empathy or sympathy with others; a new playfulness, a greater tolerance for strong emotion, a greater capacity for intimacy, an enhanced appreciation of individual differences among people, a broader perspective on life, and so on. Similarly, the patient's way of relating to the analyst may help diminish neurotic traits such as judgmentalness, perfectionism, fear of the unfamiliar, and similar defensive adaptations.

Patients come to therapy because they hurt, don't know why; and, however ambivalently, they want assistance in understanding and working through their inner conflicts and resolving their difficulties in living. They come to us for help, not to treat our neuroses and narcissistic ways. Nevertheless, during the coparticipant process of jointly exploring the patient's problems, the patient and analyst inevitably in the living through process, instruct one another about their respective (unconscious) potentials and possibilities for a fuller life and richer being. In this sense, Karl Jaspers's (1963) overstated comment that the fate of the patient is the analyst rings true. For the coparticipant analyst, the opposite rings true too: the fate of the analyst is the patient, at least to some extent.

Although the therapeutic focus in analysis is on the factors affecting psychoanalytic changes in the patient, the living through process also benefits the analyst. In this sense, living through and the personal relationship serve as a therapeutic counterbalance to the coparticipants' enmeshment in transference-countertransference engagements. The analyst's nonverbal attitude or way of being (as noted, for example, in his or her tone of voice, rhythm of voice and movement, postural tension, clinical manner, etc.) informs the patient about previously unknown or overlooked possibilities for relatedness and reveals his or her unconscious view of the patient and his or her potentials for intimacy and fulfillment. Similarly, the patient nonverbally conveys and communicates the same to the analyst. The living through process is curatively pivotal in the analysis of core preverbal difficulties and deficits for patient and analyst alike. This alogical, parataxic, and unconscious process, particularly in its direct relational form, can be instrumental in the repair of analysts', as well as patients', pervasive and deep unresolved feelings of inadequacy or unworthiness—of being unacceptable and irremediably flawed.

What takes place relationally between the analyst and his or her patient in the living through process experientially informs both of them about their specific interpersonal difficulties and personal possibilities, and over time this can lead to a restructuring of both the patient's and the analyst's psyches.

THE RELATIONSHIP-INTERPRETATION CONTROVERSY: A NOTE ON THE THERAPEUTIC ACTION OF PSYCHOANALYSIS

The nature of therapeutic action has always been at the center of psycho-analytic attention. This question and derivative clinical issues about analytic process and procedure have crystallized around the relationship-interpretation controversy over the question of whether people in psychoanalysis change primarily through interpretive truth or through new relational experience.

Orthodox thought on analytic change traditionally has centered on the extensive study of the processes of insight and interpretation. Classical analysts consider insight the primary intrapsychic dynamic in personality reorganization and growth. Traditionally, this complex process has been linked to the analyst's interpretive interventions. For orthodox analysts, interpretation is the defining interpersonal activity of the analyst; it is, as Greenson puts it, "the decisive and ultimate instrument of the psychoanalyst" (1967, p. 54)

In the Freudian literature the therapeutic roles of interpretation and relationship have been conceptualized in four ways—first, as referring to two different aspects of analytic work, namely, preparing for interpretation (via relationship) and interpretive work itself. The relationship here is seen as the vehicle for the actual analytic work. Second, the two modes are regarded as comprising two distinct phases of an analysis, the preanalytic and truly analytic. Or, third, they are seen as applying to two different kinds of patients, with relationship variables supposedly effecting change in the so-called pre-oedipally disordered or developmentally arrested (i.e., borderline, narcissistic, and schizoid patients) and interpretation producing change in the so-called true neurotic or oedipally conflicted patient. Fourth, interpretation and relationship have also been seen as representing two distinct forms of activity, relationship variables being nonanalytic (therapeutic perhaps, but not analytic) and interpretation defining analytic work. All of these approaches share the conviction that relationship variables basically are either nonanalytic or only adjunctively so at best. Thus, the direct interpretive significance of the relationship and its dialectic relation with the formal interpretive process are not recognized or minimized. Moreover, many analysts repudiate or deny the coparticipant nature of psychoanalytic inquiry and the concept of living through.

As pointed out in chapter 6, separating patients into two categories—the developmentally arrested (who change by relational means) and the so-called neurotic or oedipally conflicted (who change through interpretation)—sets up a spurious dichotomy. This dichotomy is not necessary; it fails to recognize that all personality disorders are fundamentally disorders of the self at all levels of psychic organization (although patients obviously vary in the nature of their disorder) and that psychic change is premised on both transference interpretation and new interpersonal experience (though in different ways and to different degrees for different patients). Psychic conflict and developmental arrest are intertwined aspects of the experience and character of all patients (and analysts). Clinically, it is important to distinguish behaviors and experiences prompted by anxiety (i.e., conflict) from those that represent the developmental sequelae (residuals) of anxiety and apprehension (i.e., developmental warp or arrest). This is particularly relevant to the differentiation of structures resembling resistance from true resistances, as for example, prolonged silences, requests for advice, and similar regressive behaviors. These behaviors are usually interpreted as defensive dynamics, but when viewed from a developmental perspective, they may be seen as attempts at psychic growth. They may represent constructive, albeit awkward or recondite, efforts to engage the analyst in a collaborative working toward the reintegration of psychic functioning that has been stunted or warped by anxiety and apprehension.

Unquestionably, interpretation and insight are critical processes in psychoanalytic change. Their exclusivity or primacy as the means of personality reorganization, however, is open to question, as is the nature of their relation to analytic change. For example, it may be that insight follows change rather than preceding it and bringing it about, as is conventionally thought (cf. Hobbs 1968; Tenzer 1983).

The developing focus on interpersonal relations (or object-relations) characteristic of the interpersonal turn in psychoanalysis has led to a growing awareness of the curative role of the relationship. Ferenczi (1926) was the first classical analyst, and Thompson (1950, 1956) and Fromm-Reichmann (1950) were among the early interpersonal analysts to emphasize that patients need a new interpersonal experience, not simply interpretations of that experience. Similarly, Fairbairn (1958) stressed the curative primacy of the actual relationship. The self-psychology of Kohut and his followers also emphasizes the curative properties of relational processes that closely resemble those of Alexander's corrective emotional experience. Freudian analysts, too, increasingly have come to acknowledge the therapeutic role of the analytic relationship, though they vary considerably in their conceptions of its nature and importance (cf. Strachey 1937; Alexander 1961; Loewald 1960; Greenson 1967; DeWald 1976; Modell 1978; Stone 1981; Marmor 1982; Gill 1982a,b, 1983). For example, in 1954 the late Merton Gill stated categorically that the final resolution of the transference neurosis was achieved by the technique of interpretation alone. Thirty years later, however, Gill asserted that change derives from both analysis of transference (i.e., interpretation) and new interpersonal experience.

Exploration of the therapeutic role of the analytic relationship has in recent years become a burgeoning topic of interest among analysts from the major analytic schools, as can be seen in the work of Sampson (1992), Miller (1996), Mitchell (1997), Meissner (2000), Aron (2000), Stern (2002), Altman (2002), Mendelsohn (2002), Stolorow, Atwood, and Brandchaft (1994), and Shaw (2003), all of which illuminate the curative role of the analytic relationship without, however, accepting the more radical implications of coparticipant inquiry and the living through process. Thus, the question of whether people change through relational or formulative means remains an important issue.

In fact, the controversy of relationship versus interpretation reflects the broad movement of clinical psychoanalytic theory from a classical view of the analyst as an impersonal, objective, and neutral interpreter to the contemporary view of the analyst and patient as coparticipants in a personal encounter. This division, in many ways, represents an aspect of a wider psychoanalytic division between the Freudian and the Ferenczian clinical traditions. The Freudian psychoanalytic tradition focuses on the values of clinical restraint, anonymity, neutrality, nonintrusiveness, and the curative importance of insight (cognitive or intellectual understanding) and the interpretive formulation of experience. In contrast, the Ferenczian tradition focuses on the values of clinical expressiveness, boldness, personal openness, self-disclosure, and the curative importance of new relational experience. Analysts who follow in the Ferenczian tradition emphasize the importance of analytic playfulness, improvisation, and spontaneity; they generally consider emotional factors and "love" to have the primary curative role in psychoanalytic therapy.

In a sense, the controversy of relationship versus interpretation is built upon an arbitrary division. Although psychoanalysts historically have emphasized either interpretation or relationship in their conceptions of psychoanalytic cure, these complex phenomena are, in fact, inevitably and inextricably intertwined. Relationship and interpretation (meaning) are interpenetrating aspects of one another. Interpretation is inevitably relational, and relationship is inevitably interpretive. Interpretation is interpersonal participation, and interpersonal participation is always interpretive, reflecting and expressing meaning.

The question of the therapeutic nature of interpretation and relationship underlies many of our contemporary psychoanalytic controversies. For example, the clinical controversies of narrative versus historical truth, here-and-now versus genetic or extra-analytic interpretation, the curative role of empathy; the therapeutic nature of regression, expressive uses of countertransference, and the therapeutic role of self-disclosure, among others, reflect the continuing effort to understand how the entwined human imperatives of relation and meaning live themselves out in the coparticipant analytic experience.

Notes

1: Coparticipation and Coparticipant Inquiry

1. Contemporary analysts who use coparticipant concepts of inquiry in their practice do so in varying degrees, ranging from the sporadic or sparing use of coparticipant principles in clinical inquiry to restrained engagement in coparticipant analysis to an enthusiastic embrace of its therapeutic potential. These differences thus define a broad spectrum of clinical inquiry.

Analysts who subscribe to the principles of coparticipant inquiry but practice it in a constrained or limited way represent a *conservative* approach to coparticipation. These analysts, many of them from the relational schools, stand in contrast to those analysts whose consistent and comprehensive use of coparticipant theory qualify them as *radical* coparticipants. I call them radical because they represent an extreme and expansive use of coparticipant principles in contrast to those conservative analysts who use coparticipant approaches in a careful and restrained way. For example, conservative coparticipant analysts might think in terms of field theory but practice it in a relatively limited way, for instance, in their rigorous attention to the so-called standard analytic frame. A more radical coparticipant analyst might view this approach as confining and come up with an individual conception of the frame or dispense with it entirely. A further example illustrating the distinction between conservative and radical coparticipation is that of conservative analysts who acknowledge the therapeutic benefits of expressive uses of the countertransference but are sparse about revealing their own analytic experiences, seldom sharing their experiences or biographical data with their patients.

The more radically oriented coparticipant analyst, on the other hand, is very active in investigating his or her experience and invites the patient to do so too. The radical coparticipant analyst is more apt than the more conservative analyst to share moments of anger, hurt, jealousy, anxiety, and the like. Such open sharing of analytic experience is, of course, anathema to many analysts not practicing coparticipant inquiry.

Another example of how conservative coparticipant analysts differ from more radically inclined analysts is in the attention paid to the analytic convention or informal rule that generally analysts should speak only sparingly and remain silent for the most part. Conservative coparticipant analysts, like noncoparticipant analysts (participant-observers and classical analysts), might follow this stricture. The radical coparticipant analyst, on the other hand, most likely would not observe this convention and might, in fact, be quite talkative in his or her sessions. The more radical analyst sees this as important to an engaged dialogue, whereas the others see this as unwarranted intrusion, an interference with the patient's associational process. Similar differences characterize other aspects of coparticipant inquiry, such as the issue of self-disclosure, the place of spontaneity in analytic practice, ways of analyzing transference, working with immediate experience, the analytic role of asking questions, to mention but a few of the many ways in which one can engage in coparticipant inquiry in a relatively conservative or more radical way.

This is not to say that either conservative or radical coparticipant inquiry is necessarily better; either version may veer into excess. Radical coparticipation may become "wild analysis," and coparticipant conservatism may become a "mild" analysis. This said, those analysts of a more radical bent are better positioned to take advantage of the therapeutic possibilities for analytic intimacy and individuation offered by the coparticipant approach.

Coparticipant analysts, conservative and radical, are more venturesome in their pursuit of personal truth and psychological growth than adherents of the two paradigms that coparticipant inquiry builds upon and supersedes. Though each analytic paradigm stands separately with identifiable unique premises, there is some overlap between them, at their transitional edges, so to speak. One paradigm doesn't leave off and another begin in a sharp divide. It may be that those analysts who seem to have one foot in the coparticipant door and one foot outside it are in transition from one paradigm to another and are testing the waters, tentatively trying out a bolder, more dynamic and bidirectional form of inquiry.

We are dealing here with one facet of a multidimensional and extraordinarily complex phenomena—the interpersonal dynamics of the coparticipant psychoanalytic relationship. Psychoanalysts' (and patients') attitudes and beliefs guide their clinical actions, often in ways that are so complex as to defy easy explanation or analysis. Thus, in comparing paradigms or looking at one paradigm's structure, simple examples offer little valid information on the meaning of an analyst's (or patients') clinical actions; they may be clinically illustrative but have little probative value. This is true even of more sophisticated and complex studies of clinical phenomena. However, the study of clinical behavior in sharp detail over prolonged periods of time is more likely to give a truer or at least a fuller account of the meaning of analysts' actions. However, there is a limit to our understanding. Inherently, the relationship between patient and analyst is so infinitely complex that our understanding of it will always remain incomplete and open to revision. Consequently, our study of it is inexhaustible.

One final note and caveat. Language and human communication, is often subject to distortion. Words, for example, often accrue connotations resulting in a surfeit of meanings. While this may enrich our language and gladden the poet, it plays havoc with the scientist. For instance, the terms conservative and radical used here to classify different versions of coparticipant inquiry and to differentiate them from previous paradigms of analytic inquiry, may, like many words, have taken on unwanted connotations (such as, for example, those of political preferences or positions). However, in these chapters these terms are not meant to take on any values beyond their dictionary meanings.

2: Core Principles of Coparticipant Inquiry

1. From a coparticipant perspective, influence in the psychoanalytic situation is seen in terms of a *contributory*, rather than *deterministic*, concept of influence. In other words, patients and analysts each contribute to the shaping of the coparticipation of the other, but neither completely determines the analytic experience of the other. The self, as it were, is influenced, but not defined, by the interpersonal forces of its communicative context (the analytic social field). Interpersonal influence, in this perspective, is mutual, continual, and variable for both patient and analyst.

In contrast, theories of clinical participation that reflect a radical environmentalism (as in overly interpersonalized situationalism) or radical individualism carry deterministic concepts of analytic influence. The extreme situational perspective views the individual patient's coparticipatory experience as determined by the social forces of the analytic field. In this view, the self is defined by its social surroundings. Alternatively, a marked individualism minimizes the importance of the social context. Transference is seen as only minimally influenced by countertransference and vice versa. The patient's and analyst's coparticipation, in this extreme individualistic perspective, is determined by the flow of endogenous psychic process.

2. In Sullivan's (1940, 1953) theory of personality the terms "prototaxic," "parataxic," and "syntaxic" refer to the three modes of human experience. They are ordered in developmental sequence. Prototaxis, the most primitive mode, refers to undifferentiated "cosmic" experience. It is objectless "oceanic" experience without any sense of self or others. Developmentally intermediate between very primitive prototaxic experience and the logical thought of syntaxis, parataxic experience is roughly synonymous with primary process thinking. It is prelogical or alogical (arational) thought, and it forms the experiential subsoil for intuition and creativity as well as for irrational and distorted experience. Syntaxis, according to Sullivan, is the developmentally most advanced mode of experience. Similar to secondary process thinking, it refers to logical, rational, consensual experience and logical reasoning. For further study see Sullivan (1940, 1953) and Fiscalini (1995b).

3: The Evolution of Coparticipant Inquiry in Psychoanalysis

1. The contemporary interpersonal analyst Irwin Hirsch uses Fromm's term "observant participation" in his typology of contemporary analytic approaches. Fromm and Hirsch, however, use the same term to refer to very different clinical phenomena, and their individual usages of the term reflect very different analytic sensibilities.

For Fromm, the concept of observant participation reflects his emphasis on the curative importance of the analyst's authentic, spontaneous, and immediate experiential participation in the analytic setting. Fromm asserts, for example, that

> Sullivan . . . thought that the analyst must not have the attitude of a detached observer, but of a "participant observer," thus trying to transcend the orthodox idea of the detachment of the analyst. In my own view, Sullivan may not have gone far enough, and one might prefer the definition of the analyst's role as that of an "observant participant," rather than that of a participant observer. But even the expression "participant" does not quite express what is meant here; to "participate" is still to be outside. The knowledge of another person requires being inside of him, to be him. The analyst understands the patient only inasmuch as he experiences in himself all that the patient experiences; otherwise he will have only intellectual knowledge about the patient, but will never really know what the patient experiences, nor will he be able to convey to him that he shares and understands his (the patient's) experience. In this productive relatedness between analyst and patient, in the act of being fully engaged with the patient, in being fully open and responsive to him, in being soaked with him, as it were, in this center-to-center relatedness, lies one of the essential conditions for psychoanalytic understanding and cure. (Fromm, Suzuki, and DeMartino 1960, p. 112)

Fromm expresses his coparticipant sensibility in the following statement of the bidirectionality of the analytic process.

> The analyst analyzes the patient, but the patient also analyzes the analyst, because the analyst, by sharing the unconscious of his patient, cannot help clarifying his own unconscious. Hence the analyst not only cures the patient, but is also cured by him. He not only understands the patient, but eventually the patient understands him. When this stage is reached, solidarity and communion are reached. (p. 112)

Though Hirsch leans toward a coparticipant sensibility in his theorizing, he uses the term "observing participant" in a very different sense from Fromm. Hirsch divides interpersonal and relational analysts into those who practice "participant" analysis and who emphasize therapeutic relational factors and those who emphasize the importance of interpretive (formulative) understanding of patients' conflicted attempts to reenact their childhood traumas with the analyst. The patient, from this perspective, is seen as unconsciously pressuring the analyst to repeat historically problematic interactions in the transference-countertransference matrix. According to Hirsch, analysts are inevitably drawn into playing out some significant role in their patients' neurotic dramas. The "transformed" analyst struggles to gain awareness of his or her participation, to free himself or herself from the induced role. Once the analyst understands "what is going on," he or she pulls himself or herself out of this neurotic replay and, most important, interprets (or more accurately, describes) this pattern or set of events to the patient. In Hirsch's words, "the analyst is as thoroughly in the process as the patient, becomes aware of this at some point, and then addresses the interaction" (1987, p. 209).

Though there are similarities between Fromm's focus and Hirsch's emphasis, the general thrust of their approaches and their use of the concept of observant participation is very different. Coparticipant inquiry, in my view, incorporates the best aspects of both Fromm's and Hirsch's concepts of analytic participation. A broader concept than observant participation, coparticipant inquiry includes what Fromm and Hirsch both overlook.

2. Perhaps psychologically more suited to indirect inquiry, Sullivan emphasized extratransference inquiry in his analytic work with patients and in his technical recommendations. He therefore employed a "third person" or "counterprojective" methodology (cf. Havens 1976). Impressed with the disruptive power of anxiety and mindful of patients' emotional vulnerability, Sullivan held that transference (or countertransference) analysis tends to provoke paralyzing levels of anxiety in therapy. Sullivan maintained that it is far easier and more efficient and productive for patients to talk about significant issues in their interpersonal relations with people not immediately present.

3. This list, though extensive, is not exhaustive, either in length or depth. It is more of summary survey or statement. A full, complete comparative study of these points of differences, while important, goes beyond the objectives of this book and is a project for the future.

4. See note 3.

4: The Multidimensional Self

1. Some contemporary analytic theorists of a humanistic coparticipatory sensibility have, in fact, offered critiques of interpersonal, relational, and intersubjective theory as neglecting the question of psychological agency. This neglect has often led to excessively interpersonalized notions of the self and its functions. Without a firm sense of the self as agency, psychoanalysis is at risk of becoming a theory of social determinism. Lacking a viable theory of personal agency and allied concepts of personal responsibility, autonomy, and will, the individual (patient or analyst) is reduced to his or her interpersonal field. This of course, impedes the coparticipatory process.

Prominent among critics of this one–sidedness of contemporary psychoanalysis are coparticipant theorists with an "existential-phenomenological" bent, such as Roger Frie (1999, 2001, 2003), Jon Mills (1999), and Jon Frederickson (in press). Frie, for example, in a scholarly critique of postmodern psychoanalysis, asserts that

> Daseinanalysis bridges the growing philosophic divide between existentialism and postmodernism. Whereas existentialism emphasizes such notions as agency, autonomy, and individualism, postmodernism celebrates a one-sided dissolution and dispersion of the self. Each perspective taken on its

own, can result in a reductionism that is ill suited to psychoanalytic pursuits. Taken together, however, the tenets of existentialism and postmodernism enable the psychoanalyst to account for human agency and avoid relativistic pitfalls. (2001, p. 164)

Frie adds that

if everything exists only in relation to something else, if everything is merely socially constructed or linguistically determined, then there would presumably be no ground on which autonomous thinking and speaking could take place. Contemporary psychoanalytic theory needs to recognize and acknowledge the way in which the individual is able to make choices and facilitate change despite the larger forces at work in determining life experience. Clearly there is much that can be learned from such a combined approach. (2001, p. 165)

Frie also reminds us that "the individual self is at once grounded in a sense of separateness and togetherness, which is both subjective and intersubjective. When the mind is seen as existing only in relational and cultural bridges, the importance of individual and intrapsychic experience is diminished" (1999, p. 531).

Similar critiques are cogently framed by Mills (1999) and Frederickson (in press). I recommend a reading of this perspective. A good place to start is Frie's (2003) discussion of the problem of agency and freedom in contemporary psychoanalysis.

2. For Sullivan perhaps more so than for any other major psychoanalytic theorist, this psychic dimension was absolutely crucial to any understanding of his entire theoretical effort. His concept of the self was intimately related to his theories of motivation, pathology, therapeutic growth and resistance, and, most important, his theory of anxiety and consciousness.

3. The various selves that I outline here are not, in reified fashion, to be considered entities. Rather they each symbolize a set of processes, functions, dynamisms, or psychic operations with a common purpose. In essence, they represent clusters of experience and behavior with a common function or character.

4. Although Sullivan and later interpersonalists clearly recognized the developmental and psychopathological implications of unfortunate interpersonal experiences with early sexuality or sensuality, they did not articulate a detailed theory of the ontogenesis of a general sexual drive. Sullivan's concept of zonal needs, however, provides the theoretical means for a detailed interpersonal study of early, "pregenital" sexual or sensual needs and experiences. Thus, although the interpersonalists have not detailed a theory of infantile or childhood sexuality, interpersonal theory allows room for an expanded developmental theory of sensuality or sexuality from this psychoanalytic perspective. This project, however, goes beyond the purpose of this study of the coparticipatory self, which is focused on the analytic dialectics of the personal and the interpersonal selves and their significance for coparticipant inquiry.

5. Sullivan came closest to postulating a striving for self-actualization or self-fulfillment in his concept of the "power motive," a forerunner of Robert White's

(1959) later adaptational concept of "competence motivation," or "effectance." According to Sullivan (1940), humans "seem to be born . . . with something of this . . . motive toward the manifestation of power or ability" (p. 14). Sullivan limited his concept to the effective pursuit of relational intimacy, bodily satisfaction, and interpersonal security; however, this motive would apply equally, I think, to the pursuit of self-fulfillment. However, Sullivan's concept of the "power motive" suffered a somewhat curious fate in the development of his ideas. At first, in his early lectures published as the *Conceptions of Modern Psychiatry*, Sullivan considered the power motive an important aspect of what he then called the need for personal security. And though Sullivan restricted his concept to the interpersonal and adaptive, it could have easily encompassed the personal and expressive. Nevertheless, in later publications, this concept simply faded from view and was supplanted by discussions of "power operations," grandiose or controlling security operations through which the individual hopes to defensively maintain or restore a threatened interpersonal self (i.e., his or her self-esteem).

6. These dimensions of the self are not to be confused with the multiple "self states" posited by some interpersonal and relational theorists (cf. Bromberg 1997). The coparticipant self is a unitary though complex and multifaceted self. As Frie (2003) points out,

> even if we accept the notion of multiple constructed self-states, this self-system relies on an underlying continuity of selfhood that stands in the way of psychic disintegration and allows for self-perception and understanding over time. Thus it would seem that there is need to temper the constructivist impulse in recent theory in order to leave a space for individual will and action. (p. 650)

The five dimensions of the self represent different aspects or domains of one unitary self. In contrast, the various "self- states" or "multiple selves" represent the various transitory states of one's personified self. They represent, in other words, an elaboration of Sullivan's concept of "me-you" relations and theory of self-personifications or representations of self and other.

"Self-states" refer to momentary patterns of interactional sequences between oneself and others that are governed by the existing state of the coparticipants' self-and-other personifications. The "self-states" clinically represent patterns of thought, affect, belief, and motive. These "self states" represent the moment-to-moment functioning of the interpersonal self, the functioning, in other words, of *one* dimension of the five-dimensional coparticipant self.

A danger of a clinical focus on "self-states" or "multiple selves," with its implied situational bias and its fractioning potential, is that it can lead to a disavowal of personal agency and responsibility. One can disown one's experience or behavior by assigning it to one's self-*state* rather than to *oneself*, particularly if that self-state is seen as having been "induced" by someone else.

The self may be complex and multifaceted, but in my view it is a unitary phenomenon, uniquely individual for each person.

10: *Openness to Singularity*

1. Some papers on curiosity have recently appeared in the analytic literature. See, for example, Goldberg (2002) and Nersessian (1995). Perhaps this signals a new interest in the analytic study of this important human trait. Still, the analytic study of curiosity is far from a burgeoning one.

12: *Coparticipant Transference Analysis*

1. Sullivan held that a patient's initial insight into a transferential process would reduce his or her resistance to the analysis and foster a gradual evolution into a viable working collaboration. In his words,

> Once past the first milestone of insight into a parataxic process, the resistance to interpretations passes gradually into a careful validating process. . . . These initial insights [are of] fundamental significance in changing an allegedly therapeutic situation from a highly tentative and risky integration into a firm and reliable collaboration. (1940, p. 204)

13: *Living Through*

1. The personal relationship refers to the inadvertent, relatively unconflicted dimension of the analytic relationship, what some call the real or actual relationship. This aspect of analytic relatedness stands in contrast to the technical, or intentional, aspects of analytic relatedness.

As I outlined in my 1988 paper on curative action, the analytic relationship may heuristically be ordered in terms of four dimensions: transference, intentionality, specificity, and directness. First of all, the analytic relationship can be divided into the actual and the transference-countertransference relationships. The actual relationship divides into the technical (intended) relationship and the personal (inadvertent) relationship.

The personal relationship carries curative impact in two ways: directly, as new relational experience; and, indirectly, in its adjunctive role of confirming or disconfirming interpretive (verbal) understanding. The personal relationship, in addition to its specific curative effect via the living through process, also plays a general facilitative role in its contributions to the establishment of a therapeutic alliance or working relationship.

The transference-countertransference, consensually valid and personal relationships are, of course, only separable conceptually. In the analytic situation, as in everyday life, interpersonal and intrapersonal processes are always complex, constantly shifting amalgams of these relational dimensions. See Fiscalini (1988) for a fuller account of the hypothesized structure of the analytic relationship outlined here.

References

Abrams, S. 1992. Ambiguity in excess: An obstacle to common ground. In R. J. Wallerstein, ed., *The Common Ground of Psychoanalysis*, pp. 67–79. Northvale, N.J.: Aronson.

Alexander, F. and T. M. French. 1946. *Psychoanalytic Therapy*. New York: Ronald Press.

Alexander, F. 1961. *The Scope of Psychoanalysis*. New York: Basic Books.

Allport, G. W. 1955. *Becoming*. New Haven: Yale University Press.

Altman, N. 2002. Where is the action in the "talking cure?" *Contemporary Psychoanalysis* 38:499–513.

Antonovsky, A. 1985. Relationship and psychic work: Questions on the therapeutic action of psychoanalysis. *Contemporary Psychoanalysis* 21:309–320.

Arieti, S. 1976. *Creativity*. New York: Basic Books.

Aron, L. 1991. The patient's experience of the analyst's subjectivity. *Psychoanalytic Dialogues* 1:29–51.

——. 1996. *A Meeting of Minds*. Hillsdale, N.J.: The Analytic Press.

——. 2000. Self-reflectivity and the therapeutic action of psychoanalysis. *Psychoanalytic Psychology* 17:667–689.

Balint, M. 1968. *The Basic Fault*. London: Tavistock.

Bass, A. 2001a. It takes one to know one: Or whose unconscious is it anyway. *Psychoanalytic Dialogues* 11:683–702.

——. 2001b. Mental structure, psychic process, and analytic relations: How people change in analysis. *Psychoanalytic Dialogues* 11:717–725.

——. 2003. From identification to spontaneous living. *Contemporary Psychoanalysis* 39:89–97.

Beebe, B. and J. Jaffe. 1997. Mother-infant interaction structures and presymbolic self- and object- representations. *Psychoanalytic Dialogues* 7:133–182.

Beebe, B. and F. Lachmann. 1999. The contribution of mother-infant mutual influence to the origins of self- and object- representations. *Psychoanalytic Psychology* 5:305–337.

Bergmann, M. S. 1976. Notes on the history of psychoanalytic technique. In M. Bergmann and F. Hartman, eds., *Evolution of Psychoanalytic Technique*, pp. 17–40. New York: Basic Books.

Bonime, W. 1982a. Psychotherapy of the depressed patient. *Contemporary Psychoanalysis* 18:173–189.

——. 1982b. The paranoid and the depressive. *Contemporary Psychoanalysis* 18:556–574.

Brenner, C. 1976. *Psychoanalytic Technique and Psychic Conflict.* New York: International Universities Press.

Bromberg, P. M. 1980a. Empathy, anxiety, reality. *Contemporary Psychoanalysis* 16:223–236.

——. 1980b. Sullivan's concept of consensual validation and the therapeutic action of psychoanalysis. *Contemporary Psychoanalysis* 16:237–248.

——. 1997. *Standing in the spaces.* Hillsdale, N.J.: The Analytic Press.

Bruner, J. S. 1966. *Toward a Theory of Instruction.* Cambridge: Harvard University Press.

Cohen, M. B. 1953. Introduction. In H. S. Sullivan, *The Interpersonal Theory of Psychiatry*, xi–xviii. Edited by H. S. Perry, and M. L. Gavel. New York: Norton.

Cooper, A. and E. G. Witenberg. 1983. The stimulation of curiosity in the supervisory situation. *Contemporary Psychoanalysis* 19:248–264.

——. 1985. The "Bogged-Down" treatment: A remedy. *Contemporary Psychoanalysis* 21:27–41.

Crowley, R. M. 1952. Human reactions of analysts to patients. *Samiksa* 6:212–219.

——. 1977. Participant observation. *Contemporary Psychoanalysis* 13:355–357.

DeWald, P. A. 1976. Transference regression and real experience in the psychoanalytic process. *Psychoanalytic Quarterly* 45:213–230.

Eagle, M. 1984. *Recent Developments in Psychoanalysis.* New York: McGraw-Hill.

Ehrenberg, D. B. 1992. *The Intimate Edge.* New York: Norton.

Epstein, L. and A. H. Feiner, eds. 1979. *Countertransference.* New York: Jason Aronson.

Fairbairn, W. R. D. 1952. *Psychoanalytic Studies of the Personality.* London: Tavistock.

——. 1958. On the nature and aims of psychoanalytical treatment. *International Journal of Psychoanalysis* 39:374–385.

Farber, L. 1966. *The Ways of the Will.* New York: Basic Books.

Feiner, A. H. 1979. The anxiety of influence and countertransference. In L. Epstein and A. H. Feiner, eds., *Countertransference: The Therapist's Contribution to Treatment*, pp. 105–128. New York: Jason Aronson.

——. 1988. Countertransference and misreading: The anxiety of the anxiety of influence. *Contemporary Psychoanalysis* 23:676–688.

——. 1991. The analyst's participation in the patient's transference. *Contemporary Psychoanalysis* 27:208–241.

Ferenczi, S. 1916. *First Contributions to Psychoanalysis.* London: Hogarth.

——. 1926. *Further Contributions to the Theory and Technique of Psycho-analysis.* London: Hogarth.

——. [1931] 1988. *The Clinical Diary of Sandor Ferenczi.* Edited by J. Dupont. Translated by M. Balint and N. Z. Jackson. Cambridge: Harvard University Press.

Ferenczi, S. and O. Rank. [1925] 1986. *The Development of Psychoanalysis.* Chicago: Chicago Institute for Psychoanalysis.

Fiscalini, J. 1988. Curative experience in the analytic relationship. *Contemporary Psychoanalysis* 24:125–141.

——. 1990. On self-actualization and the dynamism of the personal self. *Contemporary Psychoanalysis* 26:635–653.

——. 1991. Expanding the interpersonal theory of self-threat. *Contemporary Psychoanalysis* 27:242–264.

——. 1993. Interpersonal relations and the problem of narcissim. In J. Fiscalini and A. L. Grey, eds., *Narcissism and the Interpersonal Self*, 53–87. New York: Columbia University Press.

——. 1994a. The interpersonally unique and the uniquely interpersonal. *Contemporary Psychoanalysis* 30:114–134.

——. 1994b. Narcissism and coparticipant inquiry. *Contemporary Psychoanalysis* 30:743–770.

——. 1995a. Transference and countertransference as interpersonal phenomena: An introduction. In M. Lionells, J. Fiscalini, C. Mann, and D. Stern, eds., *Handbook of Interpersonal Psychoanalysis*, pp. 603–616. Hillsdale, N.J.: The Analytic Press.

——. 1995b. The clinical analysis of transference. In M. Lionells, J. Fiscalini, C. Mann, and D. Stern, eds., *Handbook of Interpersonal Psychoanalysis*, pp. 617–642. Hillsdale, N.J.: The Analytic Press.

Fiscalini, J. and A. L. Grey, eds. 1993. *Narcissism and the Interpersonal Self.* New York: Columbia University Press.

Fortune, C. 1996. Mutual analysis: A logical outcome of Sandor Ferenczi's experiments in psychoanalysis. In P. L. Rudnytsky, A. Bokay, and P. Giampieri-Deutsch, eds., *Ferenczi's Turn in Psychoanalysis*, pp. 170–183. New York: New York University Press.

Frankel, J. B. 1998. Are interpersonal and relational psychoanalysis the same? *Contemporary Psychoanalysis* 3:485–500.

Frederickson, J. In press. The problem in relationality.

Freud, S. [1910a] 1959. The future prospects of psycho-analytic therapy. In *Collected Papers*, vol. 2, pp. 285–296. New York: Basic Books.

——. [1910b] 1959. Observations on "wild" psycho-analysis. In *Collected Papers*, vol. 2, pp. 297–304. New York: Basic Books.

——. [1912a] 1959. The dynamics of the transference. In *Collected Papers*, vol. 2, pp. 312–322. New York: Basic Books.

——. [1912b] 1959. Recommendations to physicians on the psycho-analytic method of treatment. In *Collected Papers*, vol. 2, pp. 323–333. New York: Basic Books.

———. [1913] 1959. Further recommendations in the technique of psycho-analysis: On beginning the treatment. In *Collected Papers*, vol. 2, pp. 342–365. New York: Basic Books.

———. [1914a] 1959. Further recommendations in the technique of psycho-analysis: Recollection, repetition, and working through. In *Collected Papers*, vol. 2, pp. 366–376. New York: Basic Books.

———. 1914b. On Narcissism: An introduction. *Standard Edition* 14:67–102. London: Hogarth.

———. [1915] 1959. Further recommendations in the technique of psycho-analysis: Observations on transference love. In *Collected papers*, vol. 2, pp. 377–391. New York: Basic Books.

———. [1937] 1959. Analysis terminable and interminable. *Collected papers*, vol. 5, pp. 316–357. New York: Basic Books.

Frie, R. 1999. Psychoanalysis and philosophy. *Contemporary Psychoanalysis* 35:527–532.

———. 2001. From psychoanalysis to Daseinanalysis. *Contemporary Psychoanalysis* 37:153–167.

———. 2003. Modernism or postmodernism? Binswanger, Sullivan, and the problem of agency in contemporary psychoanalysis. *Contemporary Psychoanalysis* 37:635–674.

Fromm, E. 1947. *Man for Himself*. New York: Harper and Row.

———. 1955. *The Sane Society*. New York: Harper and Row.

———. 1964. *The Heart of Man*. New York: Harper and Row.

———. 1973. *The Anatomy of Human Destructiveness*. New York: Holt, Rinehart and Winston.

Fromm, E., D. T. Suzuki, and R. DeMartino. 1960. *Zen Buddhism and Psychoanalysis*. New York: Harper and Row.

Fromm-Reichmann, F. 1950. *Principles of Intensive Psychotherapy*. Chicago: University of Chicago Press.

———. 1959. *Psychoanalysis and Psychotherapy: Selected Papers*. Edited by D. M. Bullard. Chicago: University of Chicago Press.

Gedo, J. and A. Goldberg. 1973. *Models of the Mind*. Chicago: University of Chicago Press.

Gill, M. M. 1982a. The analysis of transference. In S. Slipp, ed., *Curative Factors in Dynamic Psychotherapy*, pp. 104–125. New York: McGraw Hill.

———. 1982b. *Analysis of Transference*, vol. 1. New York: International Universities Press.

———. 1983. The interpersonal paradigm and the degree of the therapist's involvement. *Contemporary Psychoanalysis* 19:200–237.

Glover, E. [1937] 1955. *The Technique of Psychoanalysis*. New York: International Universities Press.

Goldberg, C. 2002. An explanation of the analyst's impeded curiosity. *Contemporary Psychoanalysis* 38:141–152.

Goldstein, K. 1939. *The Organism*. New York: American Book.

Goz, R. 1975. On knowing the therapist "as a person." *International Journal of Psychoanalytic Psychotherapy* 4:437–458.

Greenberg, J. and S. A. Mitchell. 1983. *Object Relations in Psychoanalytic Theory*. Cambridge: Harvard University Press.

Greenson, R. 1967. *The Technique and Practice of Psychoanalysis*. New York: International Universities Press.

Grey, A. L. 1978. The therapeutic umbrella in Sullivan and Spotnitz. *Medical Psychoanalysis* 3:233–242.

Grey, A. L. and J. Fiscalini. 1987. Parallel process as transference-countertransference interaction. *Psychoanalytic Psychology* 4:131–144.

Guntrip, H. 1961. *Personality Structure and Human Interaction*. London: Hogarth.

——. 1969. *Schizoid Phenomena, Object Relations, and the Self*. New York: International Universities Press.

——. 1971. *Psychoanalytic Theory, Therapy, and the Self*. New York: Basic Books.

Hall, C. and G. Lindzey. 1957. *Theories of Personality*. New York: Wiley.

Havens, L. 1976. *Participant Observation*. New York: Jason Aronson.

Haynal, A. E. 1996. Freud and his intellectual environment: The case of Sandor Ferenczi. In P. L. Rudnytsky, A. Bokay, and P. Giampieri-Deutsch, eds., *Ferenczi's Turn in Psychoanalysis*, pp. 25–40. New York: New York University Press.

Held-Weiss, R. 1984. The interpersonal tradition and its development. *Contemporary Psychoanalysis* 32:367–384.

Hirsch, I. 1987, Varying modes of analytic participation. *Journal of the American Academy of Psychoanalysis* 15:205–222.

——. 1996. Observing-participation, mutual enactment, and the new classical models. *Contemporary Psychoanalysis* 32:367–384.

——. 1998. Further thoughts about interpersonal and relational perspectives. *Contemporary Psychoanalysis* 34:501–538.

Hobbs, N. 1968. Sources of gain in psychotherapy. In E. Hammer, ed., *Use of Interpretation in Treatment*, pp. 13–21. New York: Grune and Stratton.

Hoffman, I. Z. 1983. The patient as interpreter of the analyst's experience. *Contemporary Psychoanalysis* 19:389–422.

——. 1992. Some practical implications of the social constructivist view of the psychoanalytic situation. *Psychoanalytic Dialogues* 2:287–304.

Horney, K. 1937. *The Neurotic Personality of our Time*. New York: Norton.

——. 1939. *New Ways in Psychoanalysis*. New York: Norton.

——. 1950. *Neurosis and Human Growth*. New York: Norton.

Jacobs, T. 1991. *The Use of the Self*. New York: International Universities Press.

——. 1995. Discussion of Jay Greenberg's paper [Self-disclosure: Is it psychoanalytic?] *Contemporary Psychoanalysis* 31:237–245.

——. 1998. On countertransference enactments. *Journal of the American Psychoanalytic Association* 34:289–307.

James, W. 1890. *Principles of Psychology*. New York: Holt, Rinehart and Winston.

Jaspers, K. 1963. *On the Nature of Psychotherapy*. Chicago: University of Chicago Press.

Kernberg, O. 1975a. *Borderline Conditions and Pathological Narcissism*. New York: Jason Aronson.

———. 1975b. Further contributions to the treatment of narcissistic personalities: A reply to the discussion by Paul H. Ornstein. *International Journal of Psycho-Analysis* 56:245–247.

Klein, M. 1948. *Contributions to Psycho-Analysis: 1921-1945*. London: Hogarth.

Klein, M. 1975. *Envy and Gratitude and Other Works: 1946-1963*. New York: Delacorte.

Kohut, H. 1971. *The Analysis of the Self*. New York: International Universities Press.

———. 1972. Thoughts on narcissism and narcissistic rage. *The Psychoanalytic Study of the Child* 27:360–399.

———. 1977. *The Restoration of the Self*. New York: International Universities Press.

———. 1979. The two analyses of Mr. Z. *International Journal of Psycho-Analysis* 60:1–27.

———. 1984. *How Does Analysis Cure?* Edited by A. Goldberg and P. E. Stepansky. Chicago: University of Chicago Press.

Langs, R. 1975. *International Journal of Psychoanalytic Psychotherapy*. New York: Jason Aronson.

———. 1982. Countertransference and the process of cure. In S. Slipp, ed., *Curative Factors in Dynamic Psychotherapy*, pp. 127–152. New York: McGraw-Hill.

Lasch, C. 1979. *The Culture of Narcissism: American Life in an Age of Diminishing Expectations*. New York: Norton.

Lesser, R. 1992. Frommian therapeutic practice: A few rich hours. *Contemporary Psychoanalysis* 28:482–494.

Levenson, E. A. 1972. *The Fallacy of Understanding*. New York: Basic Books.

———. 1982a. Follow the fox. *Contemporary Psychoanalysis* 18:1–15.

———. 1982b. Language and healing. In S. Slipp, ed., *Curative Factors in Dynamic Psychotherapy*, pp. 91–103. New York: McGraw-Hill.

———. 1983. *The Ambiguity of Change*. New York: Basic Books.

———. 1988. The pursuit of the particular: On the psychoanalytic inquiry. *Contemporary Psychoanalysis* 24:1–16.

———. 1991. *The Purloined Self: Interpersonal Perspectives in Psychoanalysis*. New York: Contemporary Psychoanalytic Books.

Loewald, H. 1960. On the therapeutic action of psychoanalysis. *International Journal of Psycho-Analysis* 41:16–33.

Marmor, J. 1982. Change in psychoanalytic treatment. In S. Slipp, ed., *Curative Factors in Dynamic Psychotherapy*, pp. 60–70. New York: McGraw-Hill.

Marshall, R. and S. Marshall. 1988. *The Transference-Countertransference Matrix*. New York: Columbia University Press.

Maslow, A. 1967. *Towards a Psychology of Being*. Princeton, N.J.: Von Nostrand.

———. 1971. *The Farther Reaches of Human Nature*. New York: Viking.

May, R. 1953. *Man's Search for Himself*. New York: Norton.

———. 1967. *Psychology and the Human Dilemma*. New York: Norton.

Menninger, K. 1958. *The Theory of Psychoanalytic Technique*. New York: Harper.

Meissner, W. W. 2000. The many faces of interaction. *Psychoanalytic Psychology*, 17:512–546.

Menaker, E. 1982. *Otto Rank: A Rediscovered Legacy*. New York: Columbia University Press.

Mendelsohn, E. 2002. The analyst's "bad-enough" participation. *Psychoanalytic Dialogues* 12:331–358.

Miller, M. L. 1996. Validation, interpretation, and corrective emotional experience in psychoanalytic treatment. *Contemporary Psychoanalysis* 32:385–410.

Mills, J. 1999. Unconscious subjectivity. *Contemporary Psychoanalysis* 35:342–347.

Mitchell, S. A. 1988. *Relational Concepts in Psychoanalysis*. Cambridge: Harvard University Press.

———. 1997. *Influence and Autonomy in Psychoanalysis*. Hillsdale, N.J.: The Analytic Press.

———. 2000. *Relationality*. Hillsdale, N.J.: The Analytic Press.

Modell, A. H. 1978. The conceptualization of the therapeutic action of psychoanalysis. *Bulletin of the Menninger Clinic* 42:493–504.

Munroe, R. 1955. *Schools of Psychoanalytic Thought*. New York: Basic Books.

More, A. T. 1984. Unique individually redeemed. *Contemporary Psychoanalysis* 20:1–33.

Murphy, G. 1958. *Human Potentialities*. New York: Basic Books.

Nersessian, E. 1995. Some reflections on curiosity and psychoanalytic technique. *Psychoanalytic Quarterly* 54:113–135.

Pearce, J. and S. Newton. 1963. *The Conditions of Human Growth*. New York: Citadel Press.

Popper, K. 1965. *Conjectures and Refutations: The Growth of Scientific Knowledge*. London: Harper.

———. 1968. *The Logic of Scientific Discovery*. New York: Basic Books.

Racker, H. 1968. *Transference and Countertransference*. New York: International Universities Press.

Reik, T. [1933] 1976. New ways in psychoanalysis. In M. Bergmann and F. Hartman, eds., *The Evolution of Psychoanalytic Technique*, pp. 370–382. New York: Basic Books.

Renik, O. 1993. Analytic interaction: Conceptualizing technique in light of the analyst's irreducible subjectivity. *Psychoanalytic Quarterly* 62:553–571.

———. 2000. Benjamin Wolstein. *Contemporary Psychoanalysis* 36:231–253.

Rogers, C. A. 1951. *Client-Centered Therapy*. Boston: Houghton.

———. 1961. *On Becoming a Person*. Boston: Houghton Mifflin.

Sampson, H. 1992. The role of "real" experience in psychopathology and treatment. *Psychoanalytic Dialogues* 2:509–528.

Salzman, L. 1980. *Treatment of the obsessional personality*. New York: Jason Aronson.

Sandler, J. 1976. Countertransference and role-responsiveness. *International Review of Psycho-Analysis* 3:43–47.

Schachtel, E. 1959. *Metamorphosis*. New York: Basic Books.

Schecter, D. E. 1973. On the emergence of human relatedness. In E. G. Witenberg, ed., *Interpersonal Explorations in Psychoanalysis*, pp. 17–39. New York: Basic Books.

———. 1978. Attachment, detachment, and psychoanalytic therapy. In E. G. Witenberg, ed., *Interpersonal Psychoanalysis: New Directions*, pp. 81–104. New York: Gardner Press.

Searles, H. F. 1965. *Collected Papers on Schizophrenia and Related Subjects*. New York: International Universities Press.

———. 1979. *Countertransference and Related Subjects: Selected Papers*. New York: International Universities Press.

Shaw, D. 2003. On the therapeutic action of analytic love. *Contemporary Psychoanalysis* 39:251–278.

Singer, E. 1965. *Key Concepts in Psychotherapy*. New York: Random House.

Stanton, M. 1991. *Sandor Ferenczi: Rediscovering Active Intervention*. Hillsdale, N.J.: Aronson.

Stern, D. B. 1992. Commentary on constructivism in clinical psychoanalysis. *Psychoanalytic Dialogues* 2:331–363.

———. 1997. *Unformulated Experience*. Hillsdale, N.J.: The Analytic Press.

———. 2002. Language and the nonverbal as unity. *Contemporary Psychoanalysis* 38:515–525.

Stern, D. N. 1985. *The Interpersonal World of the Infant*. New York: Basic Books.

Stolorow, R., B. Brandchaft, and G. Atwood. 1987. *Psychoanalytic Treatment: An Intersubjective Approach*. Hillsdale, N.J.: The Analytic Press.

Stolorow, R. and G. Atwood. 1992. *Contexts of Being: The Intersubjective Foundations of Psychological Life*. Hillsdale, N.J.: The Analytic Press.

Stolorow, R., G. Atwood, and B. Brandchaft, eds. 1994. *The Intersubjective Perspective*. Northvale, N.J.: Aronson.

Stone, L. 1961. *The Psychoanalytic Situation*. New York: International Universities Press.

———. 1981. Notes on the noninterpretive elements in the psychoanalytic situation and process. *Journal of the American Psychoanalytic Association* 29:89–118.

Strachey, L. 1937. The nature of the therapeutic action of psychoanalysis. *International Journal of Psycho-Analysis* 15:27–159.

Sullivan, H. S. 1940. *Conceptions of Modern Psychiatry*. New York: Norton.

———. 1949. The theory of anxiety and the nature of psychotherapy. *Psychiatry* 17:331–336.

———. 1953. *The Interpersonal Theory of Psychiatry*. New York: Norton.

———. 1954. *The Psychiatric Interview*. Edited by H. S. Perry, and M. L. Gavel. New York: Norton.

———. 1956. *Clinical Studies*. New York: Norton.

Tauber, E. S. 1954. Exploring the therapeutic use of countertransference data. *Psychiatry* 17:331–336.

———. 1979. Countertransference reexamined. In L. Epstein and A. H. Feiner, eds., *Countertransference: The Therapist's Contribution to Treatment*, pp. 59–69. New York: Jason Aronson.

Tauber, E. S. and M. Green. 1959. *Prelogical Experience*. New York: Basic Books.

Tenzer, A. 1983. Piaget and psychoanalysis: Some reflections on insight. *Contemporary Psychoanalysis* 19:319–339.

———. 1987. Grandiosity and its discontents. *Contemporary Psychoanalysis* 28:263–271.

Thompson, C. 1950. *Psychoanalysis: Evolution and Development*. New York: Grove Press.

———. 1956. The role of the analyst's personality in therapy. *Journal of Psychotherapy* 10:347–359.

———. 1958. *Interpersonal Psychoanalysis: Selected Papers*. Edited by M. Green. New York: Basic Books.

White, R. W. 1959. Motivation reconsidered: The concept of competence. *Psychological Bulletin* 66:297–333.

Will, O. 1954. Introduction. In H. S. Sullivan, *The Psychiatric Interview*, ix–xxiii. Edited by H. S. Perry, and M. L. Gavel. New York: Norton.

Wilner, W. 1998a. Experience, metaphor, and the crucial nature of the analyst's expressive participation. *Contemporary Psychoanalysis* 34:413–443.

———. 1998b. Working experientially in psychoanalysis. *Contemporary Psychoanalysis* 34:591–596.

———. 1999. The un-consciousing of awareness in psychoanalytic therapy. *Contemporary Psychoanalysis* 35:617–628.

Winnicott, D. W. 1947. Hate in the countertransference. In *Through Pediatrics to Psycho-Analysis*, pp. 194–203. New York: Basic Books.

———. 1958. *Through Pediatrics to Psycho-Analysis*. New York: Basic Books.

———. 1965. *The Maturational Processes and the Facilitating Environment*. New York: International Universities Press.

Witenberg, E. G. 1981. Myth and reality in psychoanalytic practice. In S. Klebanow, ed., *Changing Concepts in Psychoanalysis*, pp. 11–16. New York: Gardner Press.

Wolstein, B. 1954. *Transference*. New York: Grune and Stratton.

———. 1959. *Countertransference*. New York: Grune and Stratton.

———. 1971. *Human Psyche in Psychoanalysis*. Springfield, IL: Thomas.

———. 1975. Countertransference: The psychoanalyst's shared experience and inquiry with his patient. *Journal of American Academy of Psychoanalysis* 3:77–89.

———. 1977a. From mirror to participant observation to coparticipant inquiry and experience. *Contemporary Psychoanalysis* 13:381–386.

———. 1977b. Vintage Sullivan: Comments on the 1946–1947 seminar. *Contemporary Psychoanalysis* 13:407–411.

———. 1981a. The psychic realism of psychoanalytic inquiry. *Contemporary Psychoanalysis* 17:399–412.

———. 1981b. Review essay: Psychology of the self and immediate experience. *Contemporary Psychoanalysis* 17:136–143.

———. 1981c. A historical note on Erich Fromm. *Contemporary Psychoanalysis* 17:41–45.

———. 1981d. The psychic realism of psychoanalytic inquiry. *Contemporary Psychoanalysis* 17:595–606.

———. 1983a. Transference and resistance as psychic experience. *Contemporary Psychoanalysis* 19:276–294.

———. 1983b. The pluralism of perspectives on countertransference. *Contemporary Psychoanalysis* 19:506–521.

———. 1985. Self-knowledge through immediate experience. *Contemporary Psychoanalysis* 21:617–625.

———. 1987. Experience, interpretation, self-knowledge. *Contemporary Psychoanalysis* 23:329–349.

———. 1988. The pluralism of perspectives on countertransference. In B. Wolstein, ed., *Essential Papers on Countertransference*, pp. 339–353. New York: New York University Press.

———. 1997. The first direct analysis of transference and countertransference. *Psychoanalytic Inquiry* 17:505–521.

Zucker, H. 1967. *Problems of Psychotherapy*. New York: Free Press.

Index

Abrams, S., 60
abstinence, 46
acting out, 102, 122, 124, 155
adultilization, fallacy of, 178
agency, 25, 221*n1*
agent, self as, 70
Alexander, Franz, 10, 37, 48, 202, 207, 214
alienation, 116–18
aliveness, psychological, 155–68; clinical innocence in, 160–62; defined, 156–57; fallibility in, 164; solitariness in, 162–63; spontaneity in, 164–65; therapeutic curiosity and, 158–60
allocentric attitude, 161
Allport, Gordon, 70
allusion, 191
Altman, N., 215
analyst: as active participant, 54; countertransference and analytic working space, 175–79; "living through" benefits to, 212; omnipotent strivings in, 176; as participant-observer, 50; patient as copartner with, 15–16, 29–30, 63, 93, 129–30; personality of, 203; prescriptive, 127–28; self-revelation of, 203, 209–210
analytic situation: anonymity in, 42; interpersonal fields in, 15, 22, 50–53, 63; neutrality in, 41, 52; parameters of, 34; relatedness in, 15
analytic working space, 169–83; active engagement, 178; adultilization fallacy, 178; analysis of resistance, 179–83; anxiety and, 169–71; coparticipant, 170, 187; countertransference analysis, 175–79, 182–83; empathy and engagement in, 171–73; infantalization fal-

lacy, 179; resistance and responsibility in, 174–75
Angyal, Andras, 24
anxiety: acceptance of, 98; analytic working space and, 169–71; apprehension and, 94–96; in clinical setting, 169–70; dread and, 89; embeddedness, 167; of influence, 165; interpersonal self and, 72–73, 94; living through process, 95; personalized self and, 80–81; psychopathology and, 51; in resistance analysis, 180–81; Schachtel on, 80–81; secondary, 80
apprehension: acceptance of, 98; anxiety and, 94–96; dread and, 89; as fear of change, 80–81; living through process, 95
Arieti, S., 160
Aron, Lewis, 12, 53, 215
arrested development, 136, 213–14
attitude, allocentric, 161
Atwood, George, 12, 61, 215

Bacal, Howard, 61
Balint, Michael, 48, 119
Bass, Anthony, 12, 53, 203
Beebe, B., 77
behaviorism, 82
Berlyne, Robert, 82, 160
Bollas, Christopher, 60
Bonime, Walter, 111, 124
Brandchaft, B., 12, 61, 215
Brenner, C., 10
Bridgman, Percy, 79
Bromberg, P. M., 203
Bruner, Jerome, 82

change, fear of, 80

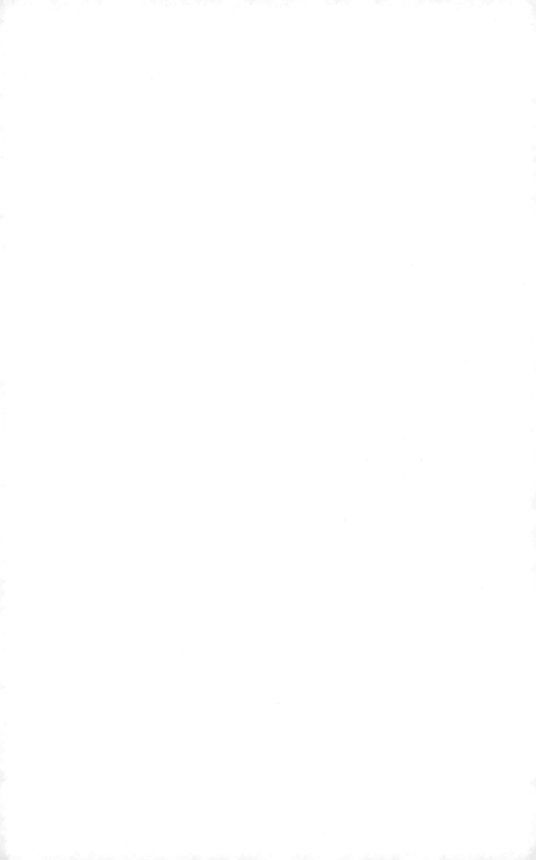